Office of Healthy Homes and Lead
Hazard Control
451 Seventh St., SW, Room 8236
Washington, DC 20410
(202)-755-1785

www.hud.gov/offices/healthyhomes

www.reeusda.gov

www.uwex.edu/healthyhome

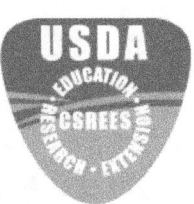

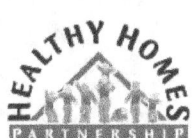

University of Wisconsin
303 Hiram Smith Hall
Madison, WI 53706
608-262-0024 • Fax: 608-265-2775
E-mail: homeasys@uwex.edu
www.uwex.edu/healthyhome/

Help Yourself to a **Healthy Home**

You want to take good care of your family. You try to eat healthy foods. You take your children to the doctor for regular checkups. You try your best to protect your family from accidents and illness. You want to live in a safe neighborhood and home.

But did you know your home might have hidden dangers to your children's health? Ask yourself:

- Is the air in your home clean and healthy?
- Do your children have breathing problems, like asthma?
- Is someone in your home allergic to mold?
- Do you know the signs of carbon monoxide poisoning?
- Is there lead anywhere in your home?
- Is your tap water safe to drink?
- Do you have household products with chemicals in them that can make you sick?
- Do you use bug spray or other products to keep away pests?
- Do you keep poisons where your children can reach them?

The answers to questions like these will help you learn if your home is safe and healthy. This booklet will make it easier to answer these and other important questions about your home and how you live in it. It will also give you ideas about how to protect your children's health. It is up to you to make sure your home is a healthy home, but there are lots of places to go for help.

Table of Contents

Why *Should You* Be Concerned?

Some of the most serious health problems for children may start at home. This booklet explains some of these health concerns and what you can do about them.

Most people spend over 90% of their time indoors.

Indoor Air Quality

Is the air in your home healthy? The air inside can be more harmful to your family's health than the air outdoors. Air can be unhealthy if it has too many pollutants. Indoor air pollutants can be lots of things—from oven cleaner to cigarette smoke to mold. It is not always easy to tell if your home has unhealthy air. You may notice bad smells or see smoke, but you cannot see or smell other dangers, like carbon monoxide or radon. This chapter will help you learn if your home has healthy air. *See page 6.*

The number of children with asthma has doubled in the past 10 years.

1 in 15 children under 18 years of age has asthma.

Asthma & Allergies

Allergies and asthma are health problems that have a lot to do with the air you breathe. You and your children spend a lot of time at home, so the air inside needs to be clean. Does someone you live with smoke? Do you have pets? Is your basement damp? These may cause or add to breathing problems. *To learn more about asthma and allergies, see page 11.*

Mold & Moisture

Other health and safety problems may come from the air in your home too. Too much dampness causes mold to grow. Some mold is very harmful and some can make allergies or asthma worse. *See page 17 to find out more about mold.*

Carbon Monoxide

If they are not working right, ovens and heaters may cause a deadly gas called *carbon monoxide* to build up inside your home. You cannot see or smell this danger, but you can help keep your loved ones safe from carbon monoxide poisoning. *See page 23 to learn more about how to protect your family from carbon monoxide.*

Lead

Can your children be poisoned by lead in your home? Some house paint and water pipes contain lead. This metal can poison your children. Most problems with lead come from old paint or lead dust. Lead was also in gasoline and got into the soil and air from car exhaust. It's not used in these ways any more. There's still plenty of lead around though.

Lead can poison your children if they get it into their mouths or breathe it in from the air. If a pregnant woman gets lead in her body, it can harm her unborn baby.

Lead poisoning can be a serious problem for young children. It can cause problems with learning, growth, and behavior that last a lifetime.

Even small amounts of lead can harm children. *Turn to page 29 to find out about lead poisoning in your home.*

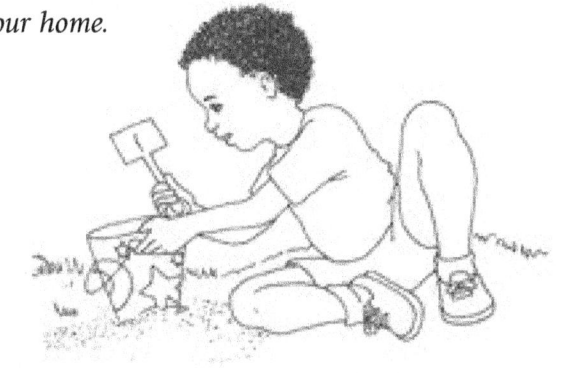

FACT

1 in 40 American children has too much lead in his/her body.

Drinking Water

Is your drinking water safe? Do you know where your drinking water comes from? If it comes from your own well, you need to make sure it is safe to drink. Have your water tested every year to make sure it does not have chemicals or other pollutants in it that can make your family sick. There are things you can do to take care of your well and keep the water clean. *See page 35 for ideas.*

You may get your drinking water from a water company or utility. They always test the water before they pipe it to you to make sure it is safe. You can ask the company or utility for a report on what the tests found. Even if it is o.k. at the water utility, water can still become unsafe after it comes into your home. *Look at page 33 to see if your water is safe to drink.*

FACT

95% of people living in rural areas use private wells for their drinking water.

Hazardous Household Products

What harmful products do you have in your home? Some products can harm your family's health if you do not use them in the right way. Common chemicals like bleach, rat poison, paint strippers, and drain cleaners can be dangerous. Children can poison themselves if they get into products like these. Even very small amounts of some chemicals can cause health problems if you touch them or breathe them in. Remember—if you spray or pump something, it goes right into the air. When you and your family breathe, those chemicals go into your bodies. *See page 38 to learn more about how to use, store, and dispose of household products.*

> **Thousands of children die each year from chemicals stored and used improperly in the home.**

Pesticides

Do you use pesticides in your home? Almost every household uses *pesticides*. Bug spray, flea powder, rat poison, and garden weed killer are all types of pesticides. They have chemicals in them that kill pests. This also means they may harm you and your family. If you do not use them safely, some pesticides may cause serious health problems—poisoning, birth defects, nerve damage, and even cancer.

Your children can come into contact with pesticides in many ways. You can take simple steps to protect them from pesticides. *See page 42 to see if you are using pesticides safely!*

> **Nearly one-half of households with a child under age five had pesticides stored within reach of children.**

Home Safety

Did you know that your chances of getting hurt at home are much higher than they are at work or school? The leading causes of death in the home are falls, drowning, fires, poisoning, suffocation, choking, and guns. Very young children and older adults are the people most likely to get hurt at home. It's important to keep people's age in mind when thinking about home safety.

Look at page 48 to find out if your home is a safe place to live and how to make it even safer.

> **Each year, accidents in the home hurt over six and a half million people.**

Why *Focus on* Children?

Everyone needs a healthy home. But there are special reasons to think about children:

- Children's bodies are still growing. Their young brains, livers, and other organs are more likely to be harmed by chemicals and other dangers than those of adults. If children get sick, it may be harder for them to get well because their immune systems are still developing.

- For their size, children eat more food, drink more water, and breathe more air than adults do. When they get lead in their bodies or breathe in harmful gases, they get a bigger dose than adults would.

- Children play and crawl on the ground. That means they are closer to many things that might cause health problems, like dust and chemicals. Babies and young children also put most everything in their mouths—things that might have chemicals or lead dust on them.

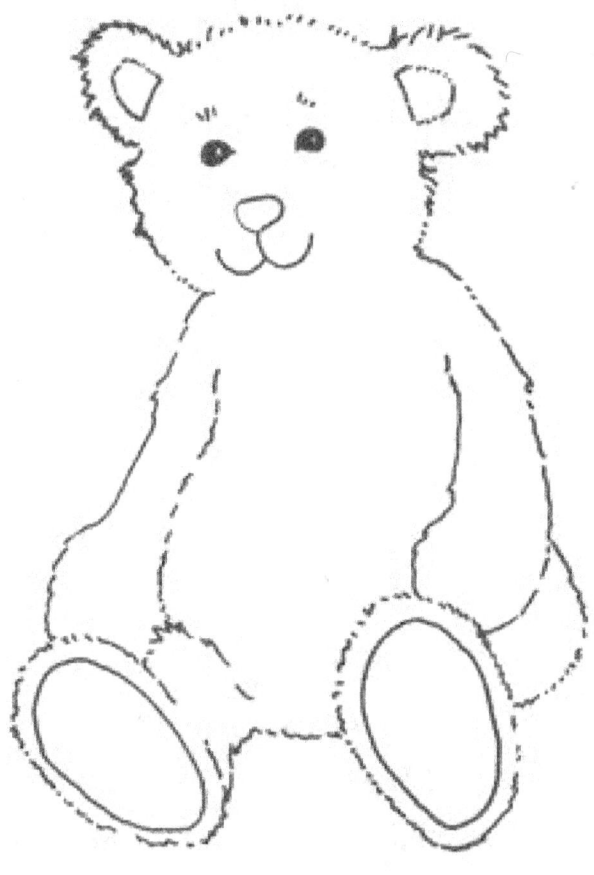

Children depend on adults to make their homes safe!

How to use this booklet...

This booklet asks questions about your home and how you live in it. By answering them, you can find out if your home is healthy or if you need to make some changes.

There are nine chapters in this booklet. Every chapter gives information about a topic, asks questions about it, and gives you simple Action Steps to protect your children's health. At the end of each chapter, you will find out where to get more help.

It's up to you—**Help Yourself to a Healthy Home!**

Should You Be Concerned?

Most people spend at least half of their lives inside their homes. The air inside can be more harmful to your family's health than the air outdoors. Is the air in your home safe to breathe?

It is not always easy to tell if your home has poor air quality. You may notice bad smells or see smoke, but you cannot see or smell other dangers, like carbon monoxide or radon. This chapter and those on asthma and allergies, mold, and carbon monoxide will help you ask the right questions to find out if the air inside your home is healthy and safe. They will also give you ideas about how to fix any problems you might find.

The air in your home can be unhealthy if it has too many pollutants in it. To cut down on indoor air pollution, learn where it comes from. Take good care of your home to keep it healthy!

Children can spend up to 90% of their time indoors. For their size, children breathe up to twice as much air as adults. That means children are at greater risk for health problems that come from indoor air pollution.

Asthma and Allergies
If someone in your home has health problems or is ill, polluted indoor air can make them feel worse. For example, asthma is a lung disease that affects a growing number of children. Indoor air pollution can make it worse. Insects and other pests can also be a real problem for people with asthma or allergies. For example, cockroach and dust mite droppings cause asthma attacks in some people. Pesticides can help fight these pests but they can be dangerous. See page 44 for more information about using bug spray and other pesticides safely. *See page 11 to find out about making your home healthier for people with asthma or allergies.*

Mold
Mold grows in wet or damp places. It often smells musty. Many people are allergic to mold. Some kinds of mold are toxic, and coming into contact with large amounts of mold may cause health problems. Talk to a doctor if you think mold is causing health problems for you or your family. *See page 17 to learn more about how to control mold in your home.*

Carbon Monoxide
Carbon monoxide is a deadly gas that can come from appliances that burn gas, oil, coal, or wood, and are not working as they should. Car exhaust also has carbon monoxide. You cannot see, taste or smell carbon monoxide. *See page 23 for more information on how to protect your family from carbon monoxide poisoning.*

Other Indoor Air Problems
Radon is another gas. It can get into some homes from the ground below them. You cannot see, taste, or smell radon. Radon is found all over the United States. Radon can cause lung cancer. In fact, it is the second leading cause of lung cancer in the U.S. If you smoke and your home has high levels of radon, your risk of lung cancer is especially high.

Sometimes indoor air pollution comes from what people do in their home.

- Tobacco smoking causes cancer and other major health problems. It's unsafe for children to be around smokers. *Second-hand* or *environmental tobacco smoke* can raise children's risk of ear infections and breathing problems. It can trigger asthma attacks, too.

- Many families have pets. However, furry pets cause problems for some people. Pets can make asthma and allergies act up, especially if you keep them in sleeping areas.

- Hobbies and home projects sometimes involve sanding, painting, welding, or using *solvent chemicals*, like varnish or paint strippers. (A solvent is a chemical that can dissolve something else. Solvents are usually liquid.) Home projects can pollute the air with dust or harmful chemicals.

Sometimes indoor air pollution comes from what people have in their homes.

- Some household products, especially those with solvents, can pollute the air if you don't use them in the right way. *See page 38 for more information about household products*

- New furniture, carpets, and building products may give off chemicals that were used in their making. Some of these chemicals can harm people, especially children.

- If your home was built before 1978, the paint may have lead in it. Lead is very dangerous for young children. *See page 29 to learn about protecting your children from lead poisoning*

There are simple, but important steps you can take to find out what is causing poor air quality. The questions on the next page can help you find problems around your home. *Page 9 will give you ideas of what to do.* Look at the chapters on asthma and allergies, mold, and carbon monoxide to learn more about indoor air problems. Remember, making your home a safer, healthier place to live may mean taking several steps.

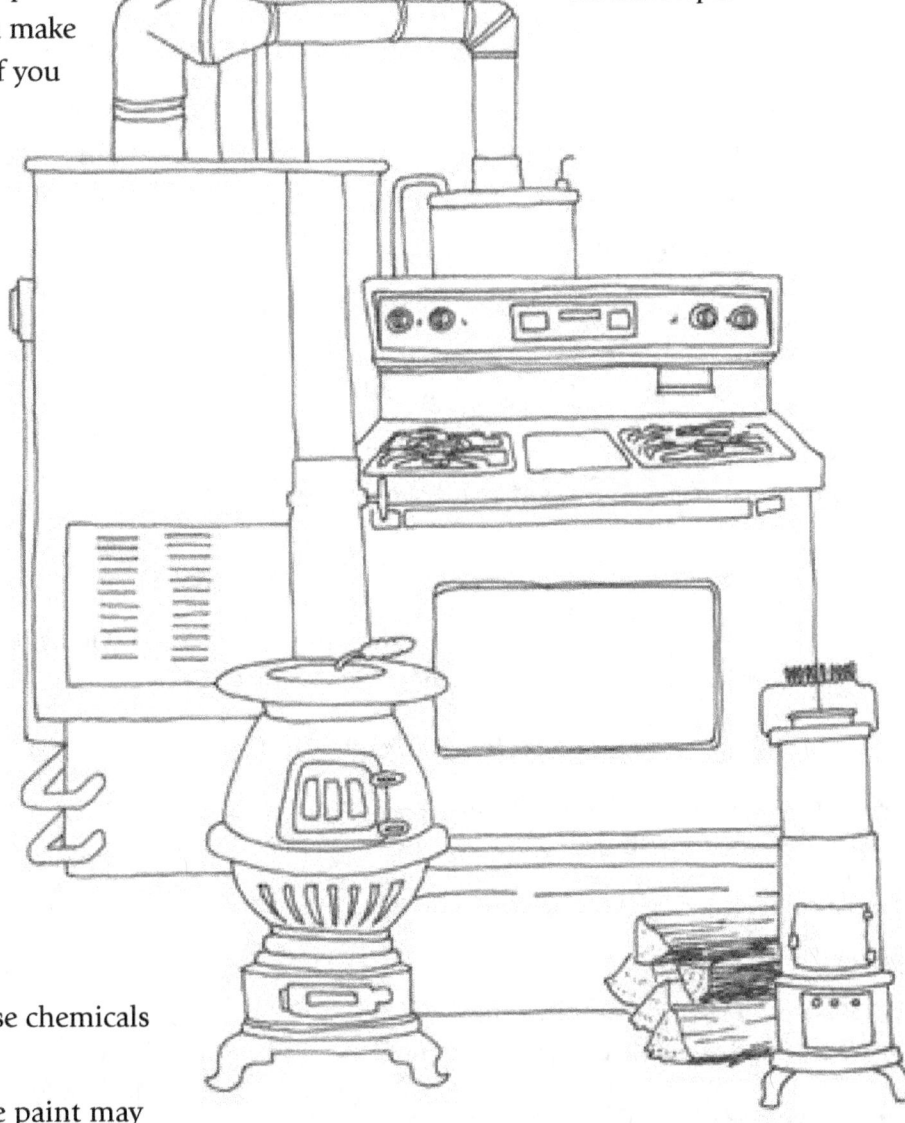

Combustion appliances are one possible source of air pollution.

Questions to Ask

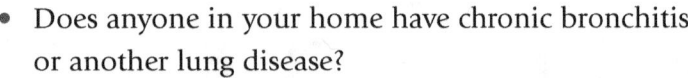

Your Family's Health

- Does anyone in your family have asthma or allergies?

- Does a family member notice burning eyes, coughing, or sneezing that happens most often while at home?

- Does anyone in your home have chronic bronchitis or another lung disease?

Radon

- Have you ever tested your home for radon?

- Do any of your neighbors have problems with radon gas? If so, you might also have a radon problem.

Living in a Healthy Home

- Do some areas in your home smell damp or musty?

- Have you seen cockroaches in your home?

- Do you know how to safely run and take care of your fuel-burning appliances?

- Do you allow smoking in your home?

- Do you have furry pets in your home? In the bedrooms?

- Do you read the label on household products, and follow the directions for using them safely?

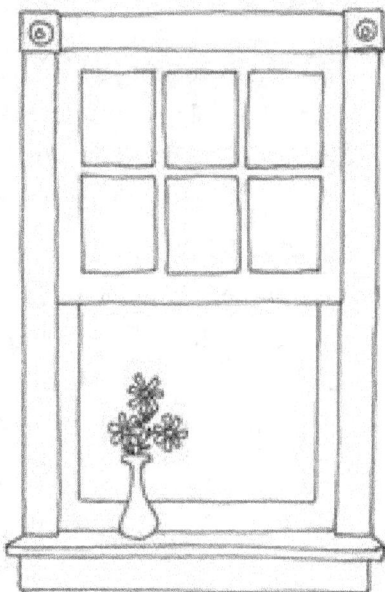

- Do you open windows or turn on fans when doing hobbies or projects that make dust or odors?

- Do you try to do dusty or smelly projects outdoors?

- Do you choose furniture, carpet, and building products that are made with non-toxic chemicals and materials? These are sometimes called *green building products*.

- Does your home ever smell musty, damp, smoky, or like chemicals?

- Does your home seem stuffy or stale? Can you smell cooking odors the next day?

- Do your bathroom and kitchen have exhaust fans—do you use them?

ACTION STEPS

Be sure to check the Action Steps in the chapters on asthma and allergies, mold, and carbon monoxide. You will find good suggestions for cutting down on pollution in your home and making the air healthier.

Test Your Home for Radon

You can buy low cost radon test kits at hardware or home supply stores. Or call your local or state health department for more information.

Living in a Healthy Home

- Do not smoke in your home or car. *Never* smoke near your children.

- Pay attention to housekeeping. Taking care of food and spills right away keeps bugs and pests away. A clean home is a healthier home.

- Open windows or use fans to let in fresh air whenever someone uses chemicals in the home or garage.

- Ask the salesperson to unroll new carpet and let it air out for at least one day before bringing it into your home. Put in carpet during a season when you can open windows for several days afterwards. Vacuum old carpet well before you remove it to keep down dust.

- Let new furniture and building materials air out for a few days before bringing them inside. Before buying new things for your home, ask for products made with non-toxic chemicals and materials. Sometimes non-toxic or green building products cost more money. You need to decide if the cost is worth it to protect the health of your family.

- Keep pets out of bedrooms and living areas.

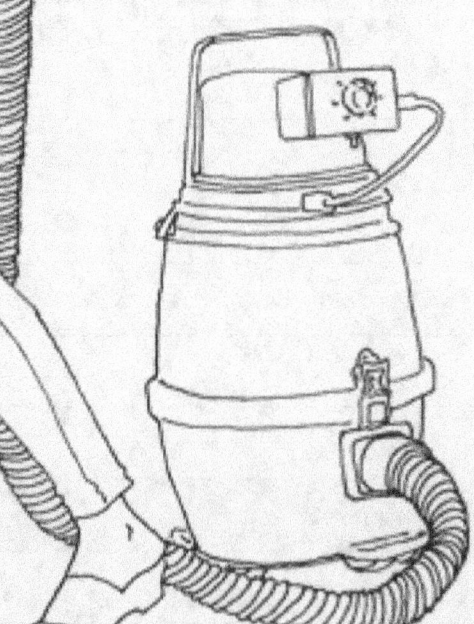

When In Doubt, Check It Out!

- US Environmental Protection Agency Indoor Air Quality Home Page—www.epa.gov/iaq

- Indoor Air Quality Information Clearinghouse (IAQ INFO) 800/438-4318 (Monday to Friday, 9:00 a.m - 5:00 p.m. Eastern Time) or email: iaqinfo@aol.com

- National Radon Information Hotline 800/SOS RADON (800/767-7236)

- The National Consumer Federation's Radon Website—www.radonfixit.org

- National Lead Information Center 800/424-LEAD (800/424-5323)

- National Hispanic Indoor Air Quality Hotline 800/SALUD-12 (800/725-8312), Monday to Friday, 9:00 a.m. - 6:00 p.m. Eastern Time

- American Lung Association. Contact your local organization, call 800/LUNG-USA (800/586-4872) or visit the web at www.lungusa.org

- Contact Healthy Indoor Air for America's Homes at 406/994-3451 or www.healthyindoorair.org

- *Home*A*Syst*: An Environmental Risk Assessment Guide for the Home contains information about indoor air quality and other healthy home topics. 608/262-0024 or www.uwex.edu/homeasyst

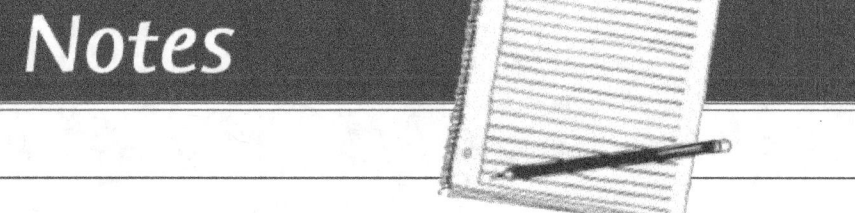

Notes

_____

_____

_____

_____

_____

_____

_____

_____

_____

Asthma & Allergies

Should You Be Concerned?

More than eight million children in the United States have a disease called *asthma*. Asthma is a leading reason that children miss school or end up in the hospital. Asthma makes it hard for people to breathe. Sometimes people even die from asthma. This disease has no cure yet, but it can be controlled.

Another 40 to 50 million people have allergies. Allergies can also make it hard for people to breathe by causing an asthma attack. An allergy is an unusual reaction to something, like a food or a plant, which is normally harmless. Common signs of allergies are a stuffy or runny nose, itching, or a rash. This section will help you ask the right questions to find out how to make your home a safer, healthier place for people with asthma or allergies.

What Happens During an Asthma Attack?

Asthma flare-ups are called asthma attacks. During an attack, the breathing tubes in your lungs, called *bronchi* and *bronchioles*, get smaller. During an asthma attack:

- The breathing tubes in your lungs swell up
- The muscles around these tubes tighten
- The tubes make large amounts of a thick fluid called mucus

You cannot catch asthma. It does run in families though. If someone in your family has it, you or your children may too. The number of asthma cases is growing, and more people die from it every year. These deaths do not need to happen.

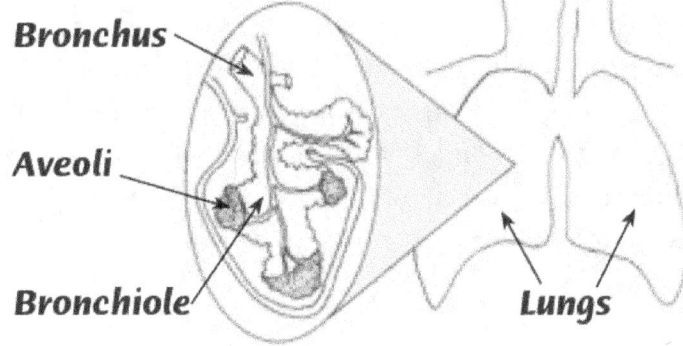

Bronchus

Aveoli

Bronchiole

Lungs

Warning Signs of an Asthma Attack:

- Tightness in the chest
- Shortness of breath
- Wheezing
- Coughing

People with asthma who learn to spot the early signs of an attack can take medicine right away. This may make the attack less severe.

If someone is having a severe asthma attack, get him or her to a hospital emergency room right away. Some signs of a severe attack:

- The person's asthma *rescue* or *inhaler medicine* doesn't help within 15 minutes
- The person's lips or fingernails are blue
- The person has trouble walking or talking due to shortness of breath

The most important thing to know about asthma is that you can control it. Asthma patients (or their parents) who learn what medicine to take and what triggers attacks can avoid them most of the time. That means people with asthma can lead normal lives.

Many types of medicine can treat asthma. Keep in mind that no one medicine works best for everyone. You and your doctor have to work together to find the best medicine. Remember, it may take a while to find just the right kinds. Also, you must take the time to find out what sets off an attack.

Asthma Triggers

No one knows what causes asthma. Lots of things set off asthma attacks, though. These things are called *triggers*. Some people have only one or two triggers. Other people have many.

Some triggers are things to which people are often allergic. Common ones are *pollen* (from trees and flowers) and *dander* (skin flakes from cats, dogs, and other pets). Also, some people are allergic to pests such as roaches, rodents, or *dust mites*. Dust mites are tiny insects that you can't see. They live everywhere—in carpets, upholstered furniture, stuffed animals, and bedding. *Cigarette smoke* is another common trigger of asthma attacks. Other triggers have nothing to do with allergies—cold weather, exercise, or strong feelings (laughing, crying).

Other Common Asthma Triggers

- Dust
- Mold
- Carbon Monoxide
- Cleaning products like furniture polish or dusting sprays
- Personal care products like hair spray or perfume
- Flu, colds

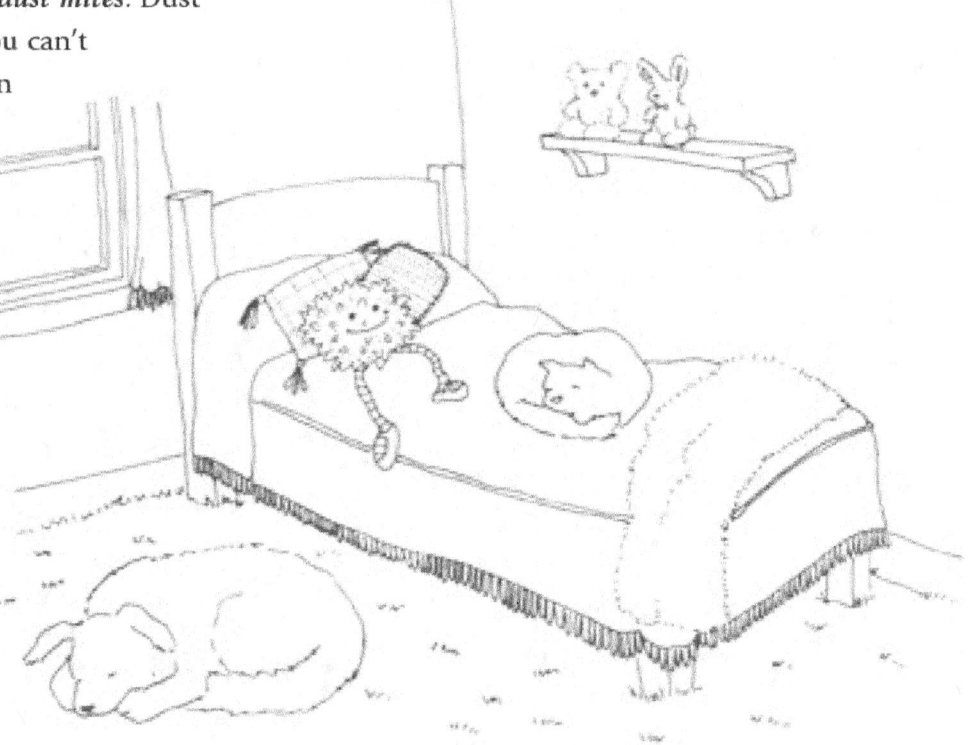

There are two main types of asthma medicine.

One kind you (or your child) take regularly to make the lungs less sensitive to the things that cause asthma attacks. It is important to take this medicine as prescribed, even if you feel o.k. It usually takes a couple of weeks to work. The other type is called *rescue medicine*. You take this during an attack to help open up your breathing tubes so you can breathe better.

Some "everyday" asthma medicines are *steroids*. Some people may worry about them because they have heard stories about athletes who use steroids in the wrong way. Asthma steroids are not the same. Side effects of asthma steroids are also rare. Asthma patients usually breathe these medicines right into their lungs, so they only need a small dose.

Allergies

Common signs of allergies include runny or stuffy noses, coughing, hives, itching, a rash, or puffy eyes. Allergies can be deadly for some people. When sensitive people come in contact with something they're very allergic to, like peanuts, their blood pressure drops, their breathing tubes swell up, and they can die from lack of air. The good news is that allergies can be treated. If you have allergies, it's important to find out what causes them and how to take care of them. A doctor can test you to find out. People with severe allergies may need to carry emergency medicine.

Common Allergens

An *allergen* is something that causes allergy signs, or an *allergic reaction*. Many of the asthma triggers listed on page 12 also cause allergic reactions in people who don't have asthma. There are many other allergens too. Some common ones are listed here. It's important to talk to your doctor if you have had a reaction to any of these:

- *Foods*: milk and dairy products, citrus fruit like oranges and lemons, artificial colors and flavors, nuts, and shellfish like shrimp or clams.

- *Medicines*: penicillin, some heart medicines, and some anti-seizure medicines.

- *Insect stings and bites*: most are caused by yellow jackets, honeybees, paper wasps, hornets and fire ants. In some people, reactions to stings become more serious as years go by. Eventually, only one sting may kill. Talk to your doctor if you have had a serious reaction to a sting.

- *Contact allergens*: cause reactions when things like plants, cosmetics, jewelry, or latex (a type of rubber) touch the skin. Rashes are common reactions to these allergens.

Look at the questions on the following pages to help you find problems around your home that may make asthma and allergies worse. Pages 14 and 15 will give you ideas about how to keep your family healthy and safe.

Questions to Ask

- Does anyone in your family have asthma or allergies?
- Does someone in your family notice burning eyes, coughing, or sneezing that happens most often at home?
- Does your home have carpet that is not cleaned well or not cleaned often?
- Do you have carpeting, stuffed toys, or fleecy materials in bedrooms?
- How often do you wash sheets, blankets, and other bedding?
- Do you store food in containers or boxes that don't have covers?
- Do you keep pets inside?
- Has it been more than a year since you had your furnace, flues, and chimneys inspected and cleaned?
- Does anyone smoke inside your home?
- Is your home damp or musty?

ACTION STEPS

Pay Attention to Your Asthma and Allergies

Know what triggers your or your children's asthma or allergies. Talk to a doctor or nurse about keeping emergency medicine around if your asthma or allergies are severe. If someone you love takes asthma or allergy medications make sure they know when to take it.

Healthy Housekeeping

Clean your home often. Since cleaning puts dust into the air, have someone without asthma or allergies do it. Wear a dust mask if you can't find somebody else to clean. You can buy one at a drug store.

Keep clutter down. Clutter collects dust and makes it harder to keep a clean home. Store your belongings in plastic or cardboard boxes instead of keeping them in piles or stacks. You can move the boxes to make cleaning easier.

When possible, don't have carpeting or rugs. Hard floors (vinyl, wood, or tile) are much easier to keep dust-free. If you do have rugs or carpet, vacuum often. You may be able to borrow or buy a vacuum with a special HEPA (High Efficiency Particle Air) filter to get rid of dust. Call your local or state health department for more information.

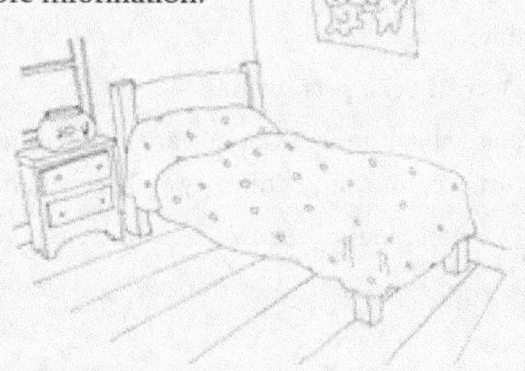

Keep Down Dust Mites

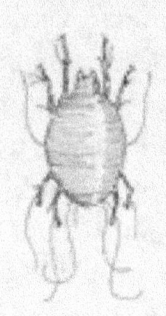

Use zippered plastic mattress and pillow covers beneath sheets and pillowcases. You can buy them at your local department store or through the mail. If the mattress cover is uncomfortable, put a mattress pad over it.

Wash bedding, including blankets, pillow covers, and mattress pads in hot water every week. Temperatures above 130°F kill dust mites.

Control Other Pests

Roaches and rodents can trigger asthma and allergies. They need food, water, warmth, and shelter to survive. You can control roaches, mice, and other pests by making these things hard to get. *See the chapter on pesticides on page 42 to learn more about how to handle pests.* Here are some tips to keep pests away:

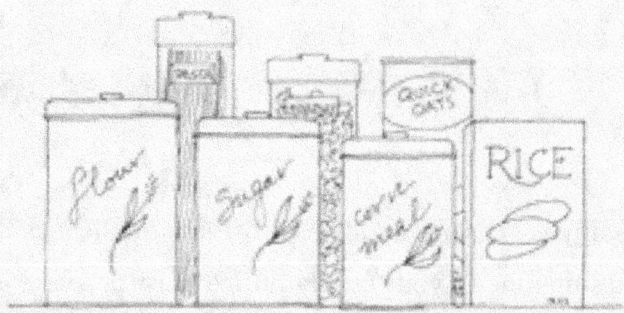

- Store food in tightly sealed containers.
- Clean up crumbs and spills right away.
- Empty your garbage often.
- Wash your dirty dishes right after eating.
- Don't leave out pet food or water overnight.
- Fix plumbing leaks and drips.
- Seal cracks where roaches and other bugs hide or get into your home.

ACTION STEPS, continued

Pets

Furry pets like dogs, cats, and gerbils can cause asthma and allergy attacks because of their saliva and skin flakes. It is best to either not have pets or keep them outside. If you do have pets inside, make sure to keep them out of sleeping areas and off fabric-covered furniture.

Check Your Appliances

Make sure your gas appliances, fireplace, furnace, or wood-burning stove have yearly checkups to keep down soot (and protect you from the dangers of carbon monoxide. *See page 26 for more information.*)

Check the filter on your furnace or air conditioner a couple times each year. Change when needed. Think about buying filters that cost a little more than the most economical ones. They will clean the air in your home better. They trap more dust so you will need to change them more often. You can buy air filters at a hardware store. Check labels and packaging to find out about these products. If you rent, talk to your land-lord about these steps.

Smoking

Cigarette, cigar, or pipe smoke causes health problems, especially for people with asthma. It is best to quit smoking (contact the American Lung Association at 1-800-LUNG-USA for help). Otherwise, smoke outside and away from children. Don't light up in your car, because smoke will linger there and affect children.

Mold

When people breathe in mold, it can cause allergies and asthma to act up. Mold needs water to grow. Keep your home dry to control mold. That will also help with roaches and dust mites. *See the chapter on mold on page 17 for more information.*

Air cleaners may help in the bedrooms of allergy and asthma patients. Good air cleaners (with HEPA filters) cost about $100 or so. DO NOT use an air cleaner that makes ozone because ozone can cause health problems.

When In Doubt, Check It Out!

- Your local county Extension Office
  —look in your telephone book

- Your local or state health department
  —look in your telephone book

- American Lung Association, 800/LUNG-USA
  —www.lungusa.org

- The Soap and Detergent Association,
  Cleaning to Control Allergies and Asthma,
  202/347-2900—www.cleaning101.com/house

- Healthy Indoor Air for America's Homes
  406/994-3451—www.montana.edu/wwwcxair

- The Allergy & Asthma Network: Mothers of Asthmatics
  800/878-4403—www.aanma.org

- The Food Allergy & Anaphylaxis Network (FAAN)
  800/929-4040—www.foodallergy.org

Notes

This chapter was written by Joseph Ponessa, Rutgers University Extension. ©2002 University of Wisconsin Extension. All Rights Reserved.

Mold & Moisture

Should You Be Concerned?

Most of us have seen mold or moisture around the home. But did you know that mold is alive? It grows on wet or damp surfaces. It is often gray or black but can also be white, orange, or green. It can grow out in the open, on places like walls, clothes, and appliances. But you may also find it in more hidden places—under carpets or in walls and attics. Mold often smells musty. Mildew is a common name for mold. If you live near the ocean or in a damp climate, there may be more mold in your home than in homes in other places.

Mold produces "spores," tiny specks you can't see and that float through the air. When you breathe in mold spores, they get into your lungs. This can cause health problems. People with allergies to mold may have reactions. They include watery eyes, runny or stuffed up noses, sneezing, itching, wheezing, trouble breathing, headaches, and tiredness. Mold can even trigger asthma attacks.

We are learning more about the health problems mold causes. Some molds can cause severe health problems in some people, but scientists disagree about what the problems are. Mold is almost everywhere, but it is not healthy to live where mold is growing. Because mold needs moisture to grow, try to keep your home and everything in it dry. Here are some places you might find mold:

- In bathrooms, especially around the shower or tub, and on the walls, ceiling, or floor
- In wet or damp basements and crawl spaces
- Around leaky bathroom and kitchen sinks
- In attics under leaking roofs
- On wet clothes that are not dried quickly
- On windows and walls where condensation collects
- In closets
- Under wallpaper or carpet
- In your air conditioner

It's important to fix any moisture problem in your home right away. Mold can grow fast, so it's best not to wait. To stop mold from growing, quickly dry or throw away anything that has gotten wet.

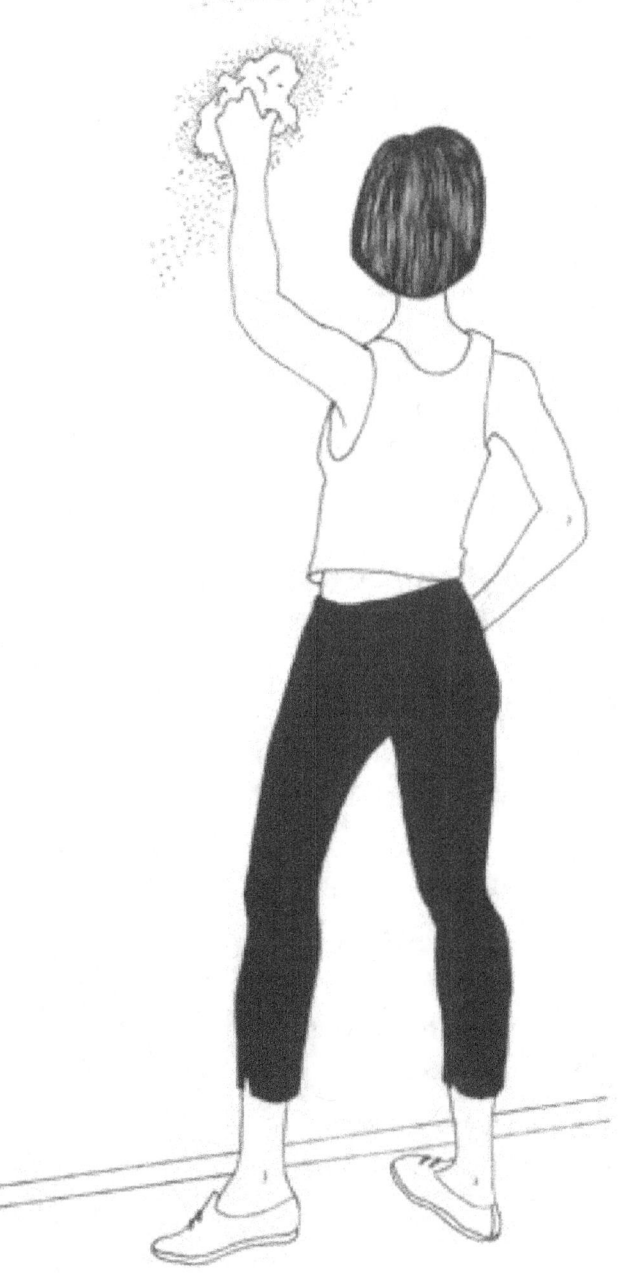

Questions to Ask

How is Your Family's Health?

- Does anyone have allergies or asthma?

- Does anyone in your home always seem to have a cold—a runny nose, wheezing, coughing, and headaches?

- Do these problems go away when they leave home for a while?

- Are there infants, children, or elderly people living in the household?

How Can You Tell if Mold is Growing in Your Home?

- Can you see mold growing anywhere?

- Is there mildew growing on clothes or towels?

- Does any part of your house or apartment smell musty or moldy?

- Do you see color changes on walls or floors that you can't wipe off?

Is There Moisture in Your Home That Could Cause Mold to Grow?

- Has any part of your home been flooded?

- Has there been a water leak or overflow?

- Has the carpet gotten wet and stayed damp for more than 24 hours?

- Can you see moisture on walls, ceilings, or windows?

- Do bathroom walls stay damp for a long time after a bath or shower?

- Do basement floor drains ever get clogged and hold water?

- Does your basement or roof leak when it rains? (Check the attic floor.)

- Does anyone use a humidifier?

- Does water collect in the drain pan under the refrigerator or air conditioner?

- Do you use unvented space heaters?

- Is there a crawl space under the house?

- Do you live in a humid climate?

- Does rainwater drain toward your home's foundation?

- If your home is raised, does water pool under it?

- Does the air in your home feel clammy or humid?

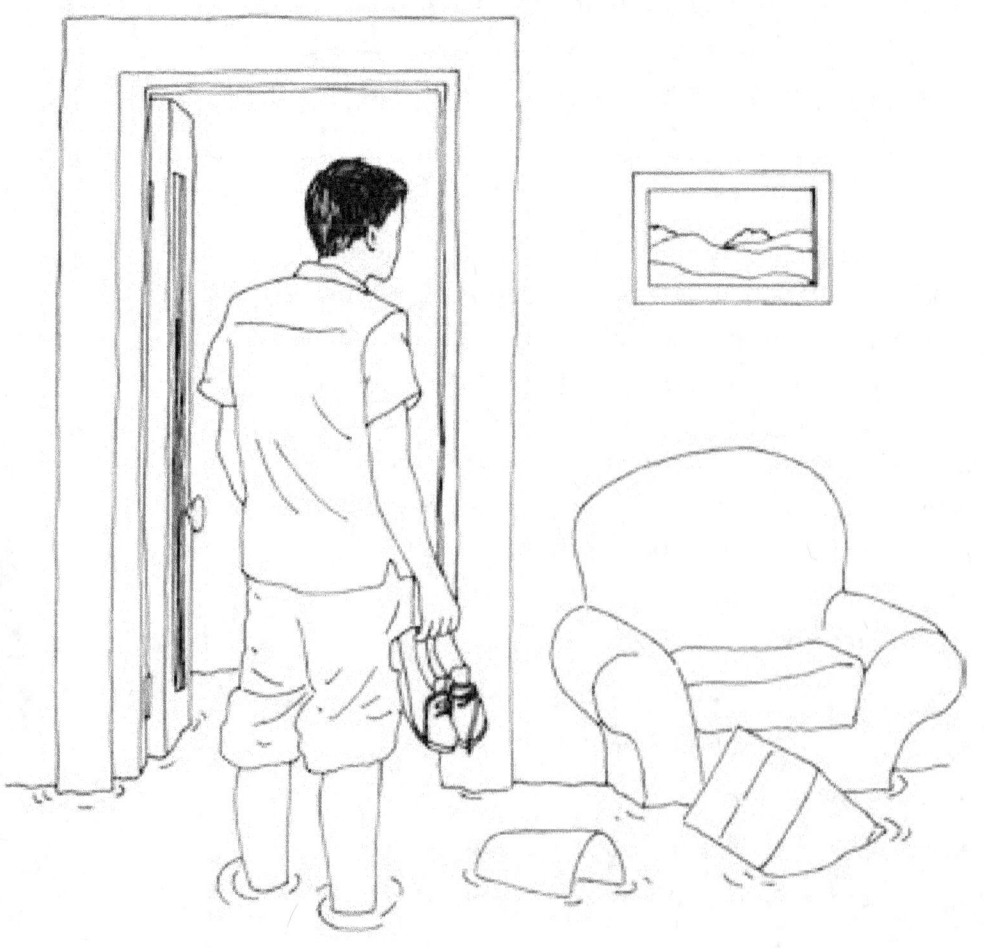

ACTION STEPS

- Use downspouts to direct rainwater away from the house. Make sure your gutters are working.

- Slope the dirt away from your house's foundation. Make sure the dirt is lower six feet away from the house than it is next to it.

- Repair leaking roofs, walls, doors, or windows.

- Keep surfaces clean and dry—wipe up spills and overflows right away.

- Store clothes and towels clean and dry—do not let them stay wet in the laundry basket or washing machine.

- Don't leave water in drip pans, basements, and air conditioners.

- Check the relative humidity in your home. You can buy a kit to do this at a home electronics or hardware store. Stop using your humidifier if the relative humidity is more than 50%.

- If the humidity is high, don't keep a lot of houseplants.

- Wipe down shower walls with a squeegee or towel after bathing or showering.

- Cut down on steam in the bathroom while bathing or showering. Run a fan that is vented to the outside or open a window.

- Run a fan vented to the outside when cooking.

- If you have a dryer, make sure it is vented to the outside.

- Use a dehumidifier or air conditioner to dry out damp areas.

- If you use a humidifier, rinse it out with water every day. Every few days, follow the manufacturer's directions for cleaning it or rinse it out with a mix of 1/2 cup chlorine bleach (Sometimes called *sodium hypochlorite*. "Clorox" is one brand.) and one gallon of water.

- When you use your air conditioner, use the "auto fan" setting.

- Throw away wet carpeting, cardboard boxes, insulation, or other things that have been very wet for more than two days.

- Increase airflow in problem areas— open closet doors and move furniture away from outside walls where mold is growing. Move your furniture around once in a while.

- Prevent moisture from collecting on windows by using storm windows. If you live in an apartment, talk to your landlord about putting on storm windows.

- Keep people with asthma or allergies away from damp areas of your home.

- Cover window wells if they leak.

ACTION STEPS, continued

- After cleaning up mold, using a high efficiency (HEPA) vacuum or air cleaner may help to get rid of mold spores in the air. You may be able to borrow a HEPA vacuum. Call your local or state health department to ask.

- If you find an area of mold greater than 15 square feet, it's best to hire a professional to get rid of it. (You can find them listed in the telephone book under "Fire and Water Damage Restoration.")

- Clean up mold with a mix of laundry detergent or dishwashing soap and water OR chlorine bleach with soap and water. Do not mix chlorine bleach with any product that contains ammonia.

- If you think mold may be causing you or your family health problems, see a doctor.

How do I Clean Up Mold?

Protect yourself when cleaning up mold. Wear long sleeves and pants, shoes and socks, rubber gloves, goggles to protect your eyes, and a N-95 respirator. Open a window to let in fresh air while you're working.

Throw away things like carpet or mattresses, wallboard (drywall), ceiling tile, insulation, or cardboard boxes that have been wet for more than two days. Wrap anything you're going to throw away in plastic to stop mold from spreading. Cleaning up mold puts the spores in the air so it's a good idea to wear a respirator. Keep small children, elderly and sick people, and anyone with allergies or asthma away during cleanup.

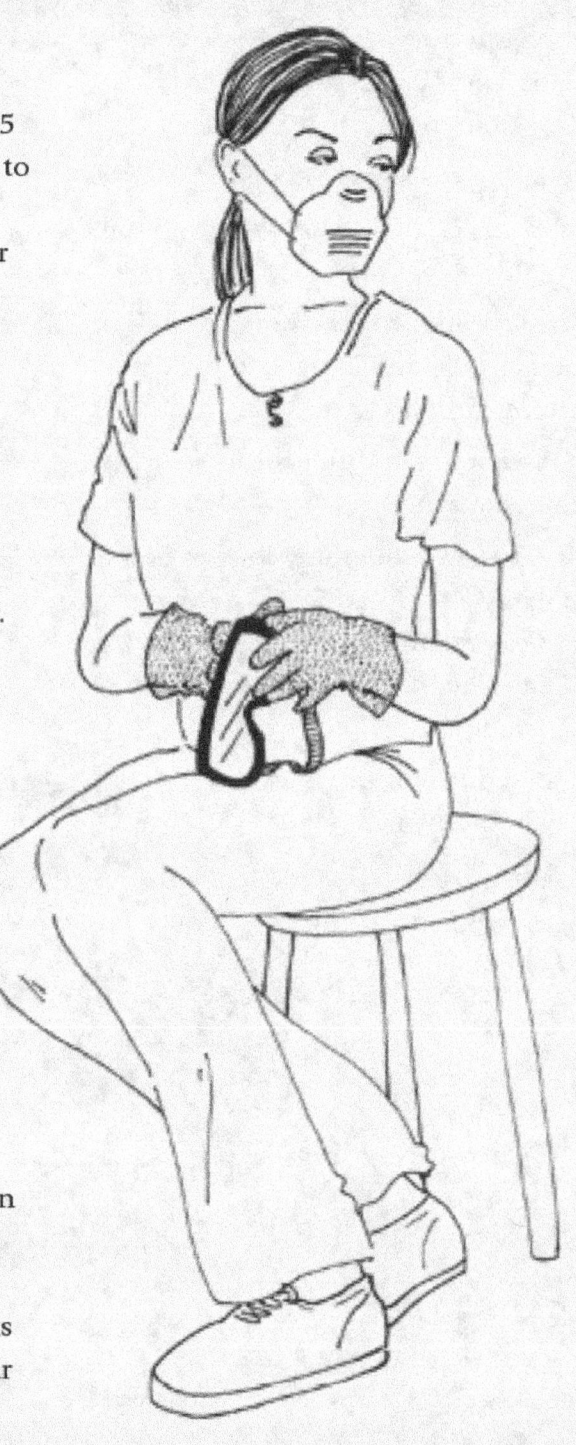

ACTION STEPS, continued

Clean hard surfaces with a mix of laundry detergent or dishwashing soap and water. You may have to scrub with a brush. Rinse the area with clean water and dry quickly by wiping away the water and using a fan. Chlorine bleach will kill mold growing on surfaces. It does not kill mold spores in the air and dead mold can still cause allergic reactions. If you use bleach, follow these steps:

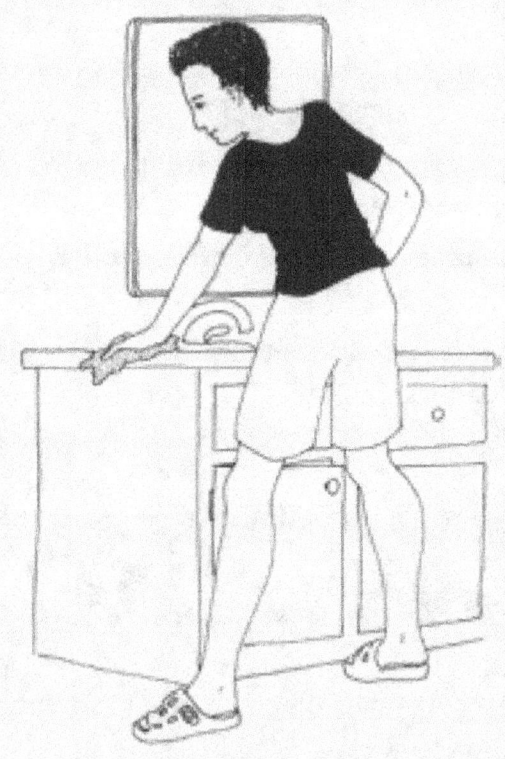

- Scrub the surface first with water and detergent.

- Water down the chlorine bleach—use about one cup bleach to ten cups of water.

- Spray or sponge the bleach on the moldy area. Leave it on about 15 minutes, then rinse the area and dry quickly.

- Never mix chlorine bleach with products that contain ammonia or acids because you will make a deadly gas.

- Keep chlorine bleach out of the reach of pets and children.

- Remember, chlorine bleach takes the color out of most fabrics and rugs. Be careful not to spill or splash.

The Cooperative Extension Service or your local or state health department can provide more information on mold. Renters should talk to their landlords. Some home insurance policies will pay to fix mold damage. Fire and Water Damage Restoration professionals can help you fix the damage. Cleaning up a big mold problem may cost several thousand dollars or more.

What About Testing for Mold?

You may have heard about so-called "toxic" molds that can cause severe health problems. This may cause worry if you know that mold is growing in your home. See your doctor if you think mold is causing health problems for you or your family. Many experts agree that health problems come more from the length of time you've been in contact with the mold and the amount of mold in your home than the type of mold in your home.

No matter what kind of mold you have, you need to get rid of it and fix the moisture problems that made it grow. Most experts think it's better to spend your time and money on cleaning up the problem than testing. So act quickly to get rid of the mold and moisture by following the action steps in this chapter.

When In Doubt, Check It Out!

- Your local county Cooperative Extension Office
  —look in your telephone book

- Your local or state health department
  —look in your telephone book

- The Environmental Protection Agency (EPA)
  —www.epa.gov/iaq

- The Centers for Disease Control & Prevention (CDC)
  —www.cdc.gov/nceh/mold

- California Indoor Air Quality Program
  —www.cal-iaq.org//iaqsheet.htm

- The Health House—www.healthhouse.org

- Healthy Indoor Air for America's Homes
  406/994-3451—www.montana.edu/wwwcxair

Notes

_____

_____

_____

_____

_____

_____

_____

_____

_____

_____

_____

_____

This chapter was written by Marilyn Bode, Extension Specialist, Iowa State University. ©2002 University of Wisconsin Extension. All Rights Reserved.

Carbon Monoxide

Should You Be Concerned?

You can't see, taste, feel, or smell carbon monoxide (CO). However, this deadly gas can make you very sick or even kill you. Over 500 people in the United States die every year after breathing too much CO. The signs of CO poisoning seem like the flu. Many people don't even know they've been breathing in CO. People who survive can suffer brain damage, lose their sight or hearing, or have heart problems. It is a major threat to your family's health. The good news is that you can prevent CO poisoning. This section will help you ask the right questions to find out if the air in your home is safe and healthy.

There can be so much CO in a burning building that breathing smoke for as little as one minute can kill you. Lower levels, such as from smoking, do not kill right away. They can cause many other health problems though. Children, unborn babies, people with asthma, older adults, or people with heart or lung problems are more likely to get hurt from breathing CO. But remember, CO harms even healthy people.

Where Does CO Come From?

Fuel-burning appliances use gas, oil, or wood to produce heat. If they are not working right, they can make CO. Most gas appliances that have been put in and taken care of properly are safe and make very little CO but unvented appliances may not be. Electric appliances do not burn fuel and so make no CO. Common sources of CO include:

- Gas and oil furnaces, boilers, and water heaters
- Wood-burning fireplaces and stoves
- Gas appliances like ovens, stoves, or dryers
- Gas and kerosene space heaters
- Gas and charcoal grills
- Cars, trucks, campers, tractors, and other vehicles
- Gasoline and liquid propane (LP)-powered small equipment, including lawn mowers, snow blowers, chainsaws, pressure washers, and electric generators
- Recreational vehicles, including boat motors, all terrain vehicles (ATVs), ski-boats, and generators in campers and houseboats
- Tobacco smoke
- House fires
- Blocked chimneys and flues

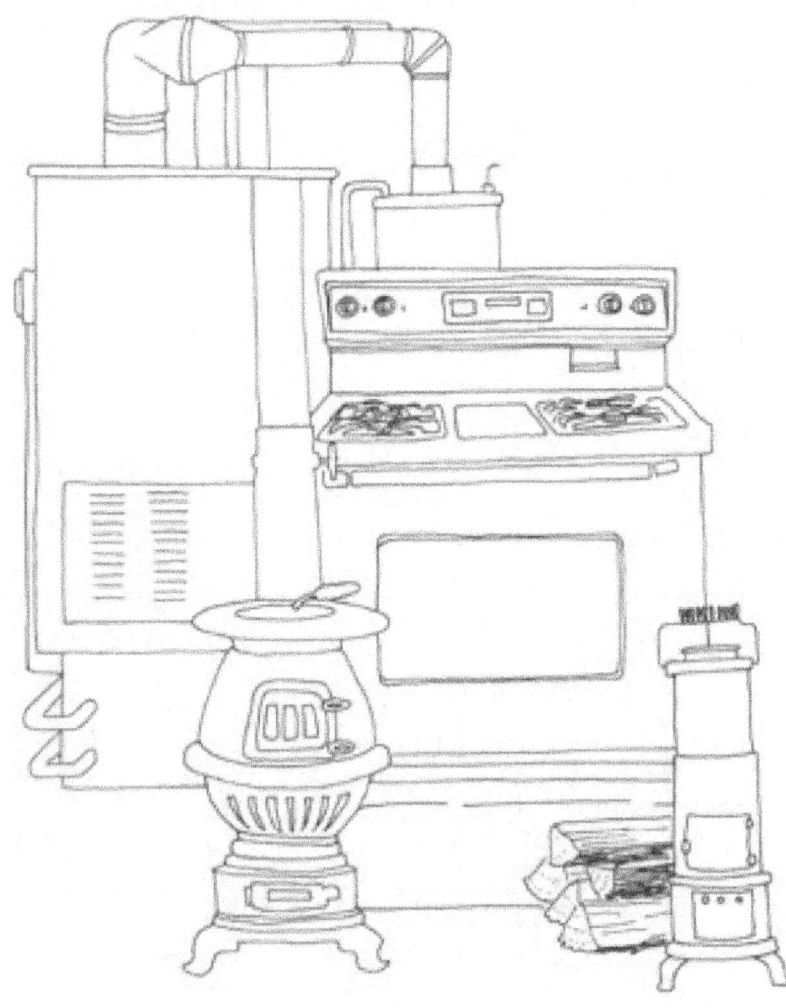

Breathing in low levels of CO can hurt your brain, heart, or other parts of your body. At high levels, the brain is so short of oxygen that you cannot think clearly. You lose control of your muscles and may be unable to move to safety. High-level CO poisoning can cause loss of consciousness, coma, and death.

There are simple but important steps to take to find out if your family is at risk for CO poisoning. The questions on the following page will help you do that. Page 27 will give you ideas of what to do to keep the air in your home safe to breathe.

What are the Signs of CO Poisoning?

People often think CO poisoning is the flu. That's because it can feel like the flu. Signs of low-level CO poisoning may include:

- Headache
- Nausea
- Vomiting
- Dizziness
- Confusion
- Tiredness
- Weakness
- Sleepiness
- Tightness in the chest
- Trouble breathing
- Changes in senses of sight, smell, hearing, touch and taste.

CO and Smoking

If you smoke, you breathe in carbon monoxide and many other chemicals. If you smoke indoors, people around you also breathe the smoke (called second-hand or environmental tobacco smoke). Smoking can make minor health problems worse and cause major diseases like cancer and heart disease. If you need help quitting, contact the American Lung Association at 1-800-LUNG-USA.

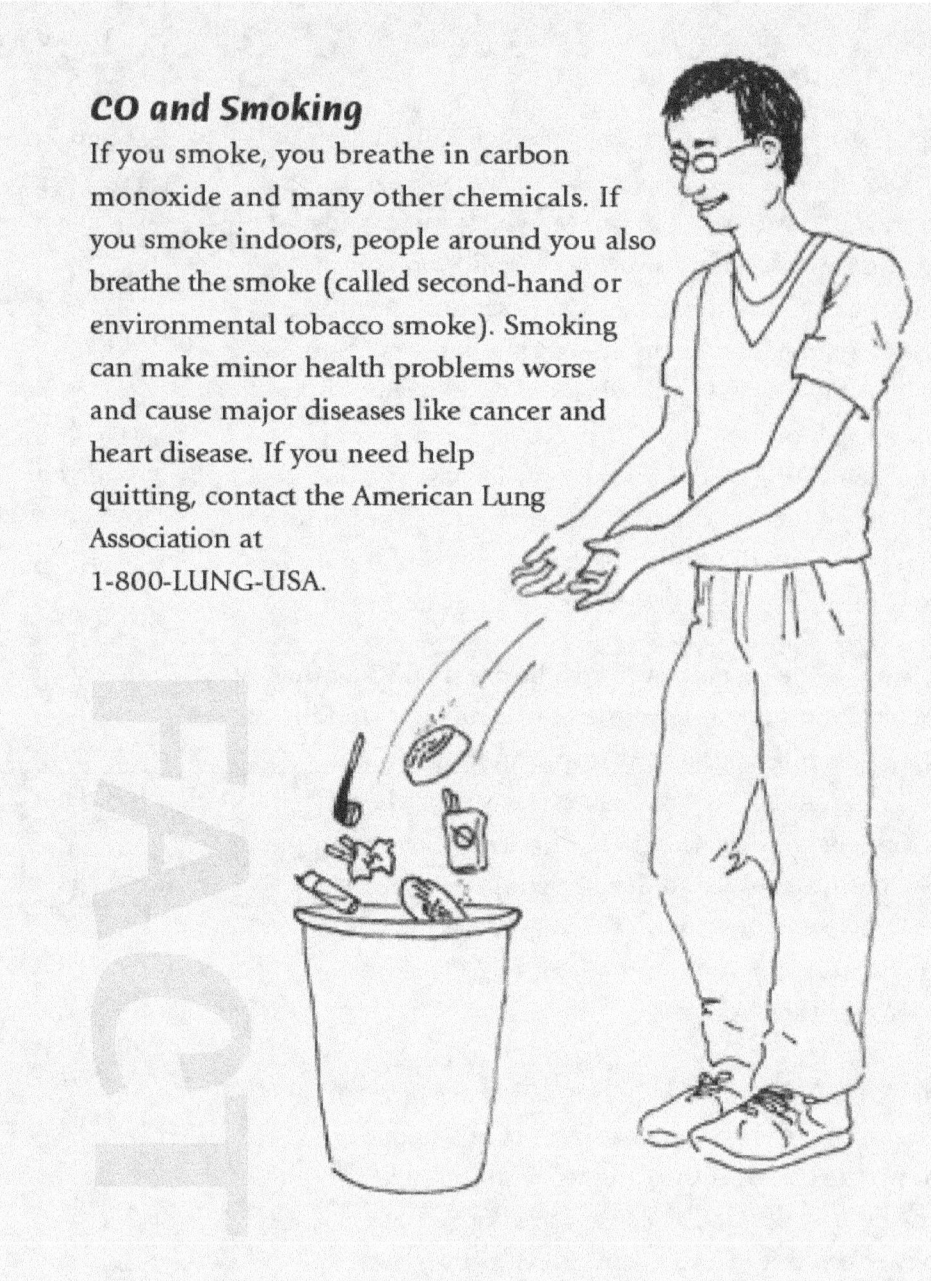

Questions to Ask

- Do you sometimes use charcoal grills or small gasoline engines inside your home, garage, or closed-in porch?

- Do you have an attached garage?

- Do you sometimes warm up your car inside the garage?

- Has it been more than one year since you or your landlord had your furnace, fireplace, wood stove, chimney or other appliances inspected or cleaned?

- Do you ever use a gas or kerosene space heater or a vent-free gas fireplace?

- Does your home have a carbon monoxide alarm?

- Do you ever use the kitchen stove or oven to heat your home?

- Do you sometimes forget to turn on the kitchen exhaust fan when using the oven?

- Do some of the burners on the kitchen stove burn yellow or orange?*

- Does smoke from the fireplace sometimes come back into the room?

- Are your appliances and furnace in good shape?

- Are the vent pipes for your furnace, boiler, or water heater rusty or falling apart?*

- Do you have a gas water heater that does not have a vent?*

- Is there rust, soot, or dirt on your furnace, boiler, or water heater?*

- Is your furnace or boiler over ten years old?*

- Have you weather-stripped doors and windows or insulated your home?*

- Have you closed off vent or combustion air openings?*

See the Safety Checklist on page 26

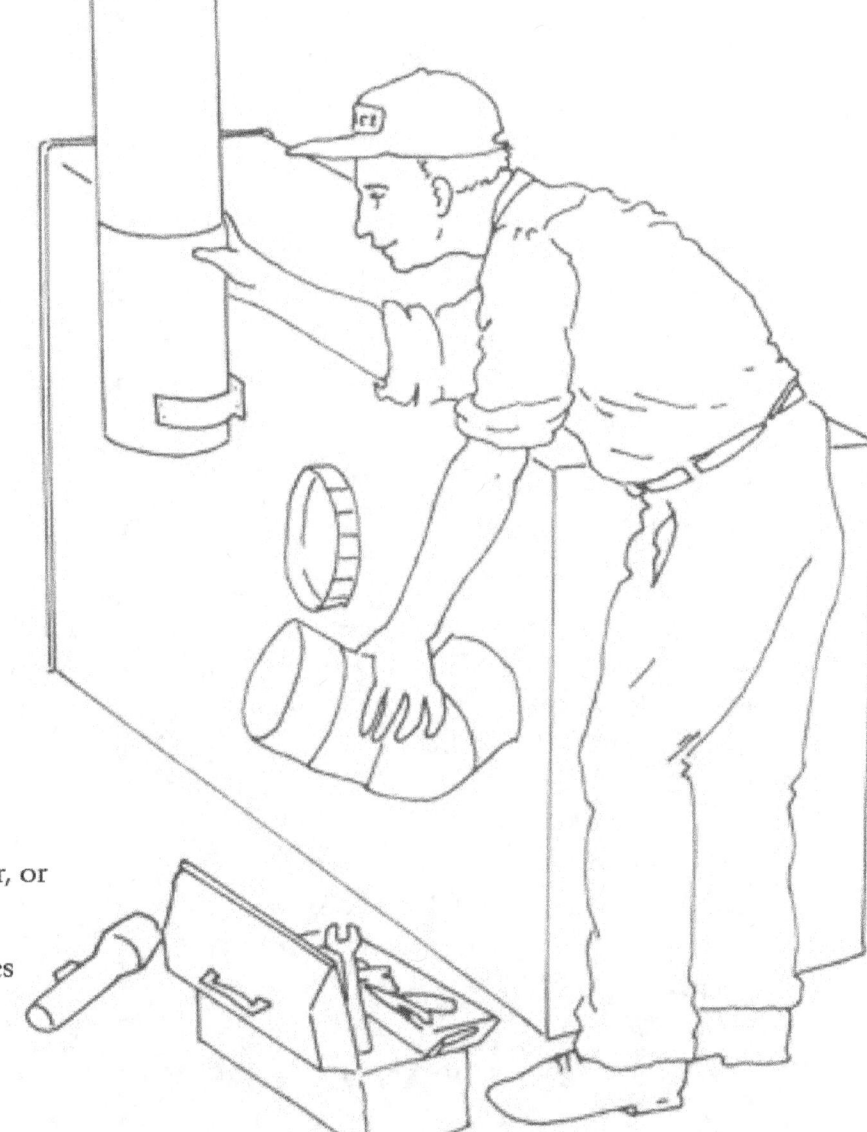

ACTION STEPS

- *Never* use charcoal grills or run engines inside your home, garage, or basement even for a short time. Charcoal grills and small gasoline engines make a lot of carbon monoxide. Even opening all the windows and doors will not give you enough fresh air to prevent CO poisoning.

- *Never* warm up a vehicle inside the garage. Warming up your car, truck, or motorcycle on a cold day for just a couple of minutes (even with the garage door open) can make enough CO to make you sick. Start lawnmowers, snow blowers, and other yard equipment outdoors.

- Have a heating contractor check your furnace, chimneys, and other sources of CO every fall to make sure everything is okay. (You can find one in the telephone book.) Make sure they use a tool that measures CO. To get harmful gases out of a home, many heating appliances have chimneys. (Chimneys on gas appliances are called vents). The chimney carries CO and other gases from the appliance outdoors. If your appliances and vents are working right there should be little CO in your home. If you rent, ask your landlord to have the heating system checked.

- Make sure chimneys are in good shape—clean and working right. Have your chimney, wood-burning fireplace, or wood stove swept every year. Burning wood nearly always makes a lot of CO. It is very important that all the smoke goes out the chimney.

- If you use unvented kerosene or gas heaters OR a vent-free gas fireplace, follow instructions carefully and always open a window for fresh air. Do not use them while sleeping.

Safety Checklist ✓

If you answered *yes* to any of the starred questions on page 25 pay special attention to this checklist. Remember, putting in and taking care of cooking and heating appliances like stoves and furnaces can be dangerous. Only trained and qualified workers should do this.

- Turn off an appliance or heater that starts making different noises, smells funny, starts sooting, has a yellow or orange-colored flame, or does not seem to be working right. Call a heating contractor for repairs.

- Read and follow the instructions that came with your appliance or unvented gas heater. Never block or disconnect an exhaust vent.

- Provide good ventilation for all heating appliances.

- Keep all wood, paper, cloth, and furniture away from heating appliances.

- Don't block an appliance's air openings or exhaust vents.

- Have furnaces checked every year by a qualified heating contractor.

- Ask the contractor to check for carbon monoxide and look at the vent (chimney) system.

- If you insulate and weather-strip your home, call a heating contractor to make sure there is still enough ventilation.

- If you smell gas or if the smoke detector or the carbon monoxide alarm goes off, leave the building right away and call 9-1-1.

ACTION STEPS, continued

- Put carbon monoxide alarms near each sleeping area and on each floor of your home. (Older models are called carbon monoxide detectors.) You can find them at your local hardware, discount, outlet, or building supply store for $20 to $50.

- Never use the kitchen stove or oven to heat your home.

- Always turn on the kitchen exhaust fan when using a non-electric oven or range top.

- Have the kitchen range top fixed before using it if the flames burn orange or yellow.

- Don't use a smoking fireplace until you fix the problem.

Carbon Monoxide Alarms

Carbon monoxide (CO) alarms will help protect you and your family from sickness or death. A good alarm will make a loud noise when CO levels become too high. There are plug-in and battery operated alarms. Look on the package to make sure the alarm is okayed by a qualified testing laboratory, such as Underwriters Laboratory (UL). Check the batteries on a battery-operated alarm every six months. Every home should have at least one alarm. It's best to put one near each sleeping area and on each level of the home. Carbon monoxide alarms do not take the place of checking and taking good care of your home's furnace, fireplace, space heaters, and oven.

If someone in your family shows signs of CO poisoning or if a CO alarm goes off:
- Get outside right away.

- Call 9-1-1 or your local emergency number from a phone outside your home.

- See a doctor or nurse right away. See a doctor or nurse even if you feel better after breathing fresh air. They can check your blood and breath for CO and tell if you need more medical care.

- Treat all alarm soundings as an emergency. Never ignore an alarm sounding!

- Have your home checked out by a qualified heating or appliance contractor. You can find one in the telephone book.

- Don't go back home until all problems have been found and fixed.

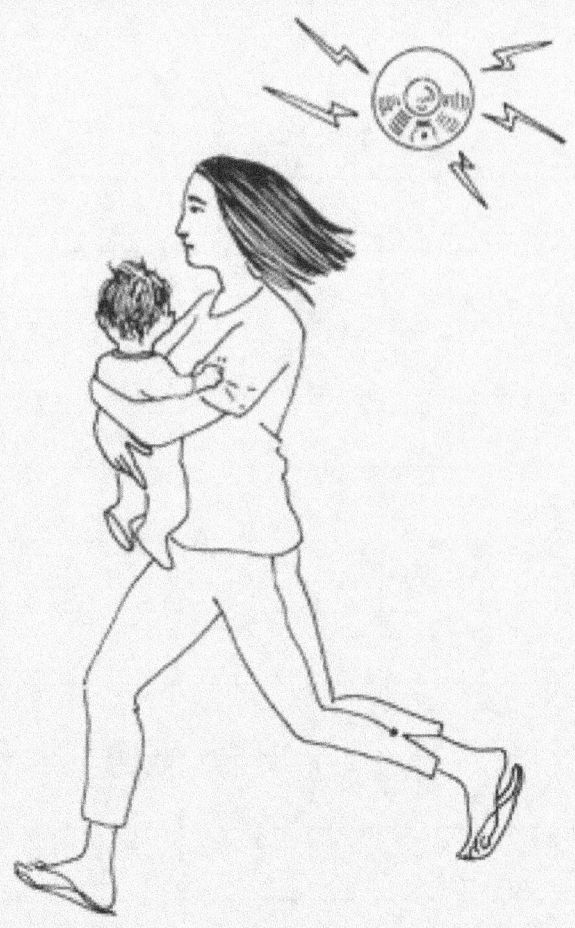

When In Doubt, Check It Out!

- Your local county Extension Office
  —look in your telephone book

- Your local or state health department
  —look in your telephone book

- The Consumer Products Safety Commission
  800/638-2772—www.cpsc.gov/cpscpub/pubs/466.html

- The American Lung Association, 800/LUNG-USA
  —www.lungusa.org/air/carbon_facstsheet99.html

- Healthy Indoor Air for America's Homes
  406/994-3451—www.montana.edu/wwwcxair/

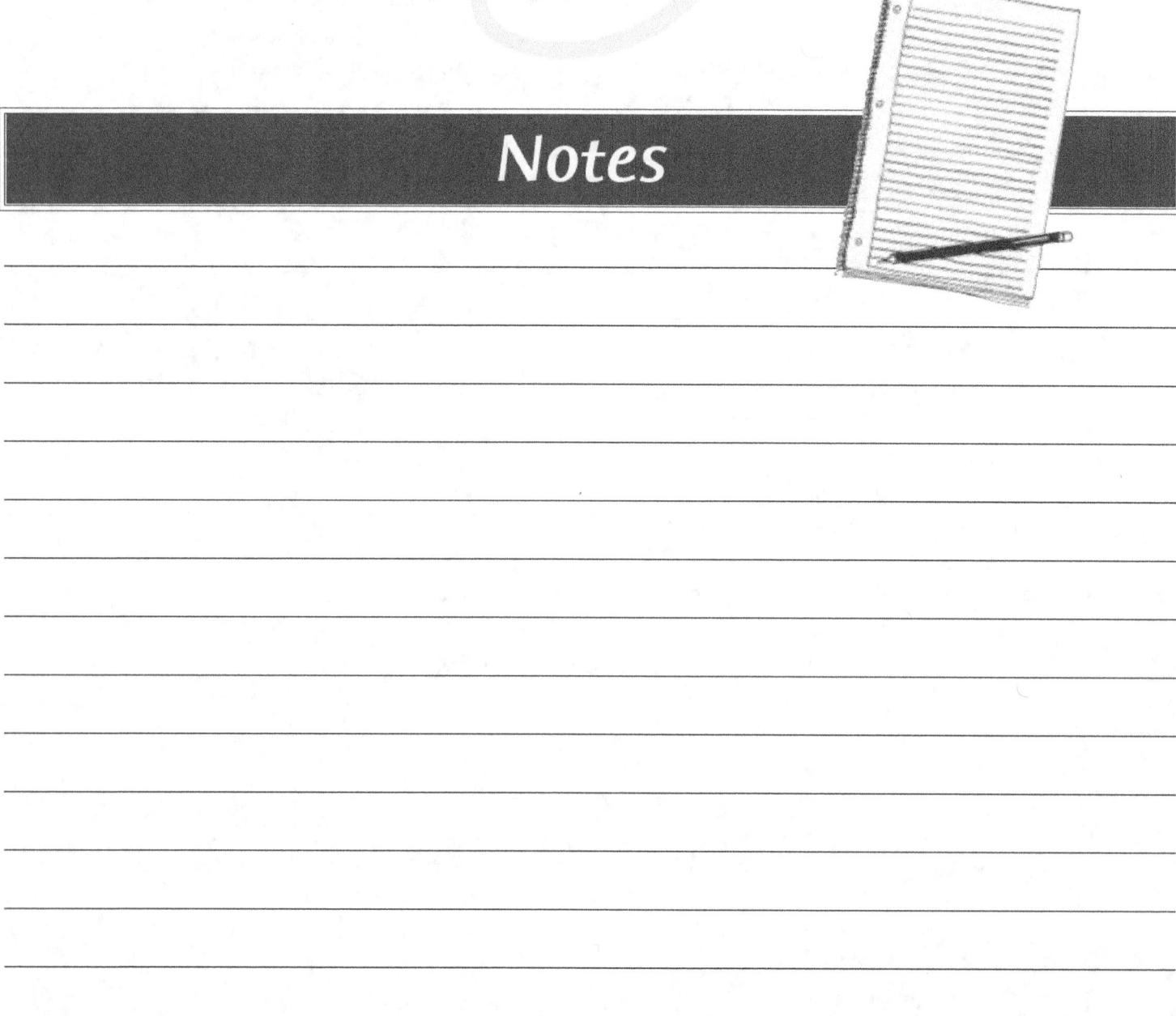

Notes

Should You Be Concerned?

Lead poisoning is one of the most serious health threats for children in and around the home. Your children can be poisoned if they get lead in their bodies. Lead may cause learning and behavior problems. It may damage hearing and the nervous system, including the brain.

Where Does Lead Come From?

Lead was used in paint, water pipes, gasoline, pottery, and other places. Even though this metal is not used as much anymore, it still remains in places it was used.

The paint on your walls and windowsills may have lead in it. Household dust (from old, worn paint) may have lead in it. Your drinking water may have lead in it from your water pipes or the solder that joins pipes together. Even the soil outside your home may have lead in it.

It is very important to find out if your home has lead in or around it. There are tests that will let you know and they don't cost a lot.

How Can Lead Poison your Child?

There are many ways. Young children put their hands and everything else in their mouths, so they can eat the dust or chips of lead-based paint without knowing it. Even bits of paint too small to see can come off windows, doors, and walls, creating lead dust. Children who crawl on the floor, put toys in their mouths, or play in soil around their home or daycare can be poisoned.

Children with too much lead in their bodies may not look or feel sick. A simple blood test is the only way to know if your child is being exposed to lead. Ask your doctor or health care provider to test your child for lead.

Lead paint that is in good shape is not an immediate problem. It may be a risk in the future though.

Laws have been passed to ban lead in household paint, gasoline and water pipes. However, many older homes still have lead in them. Finding out if lead is a problem in your home is the first step in protecting your children's health. The questions on the next page can help.

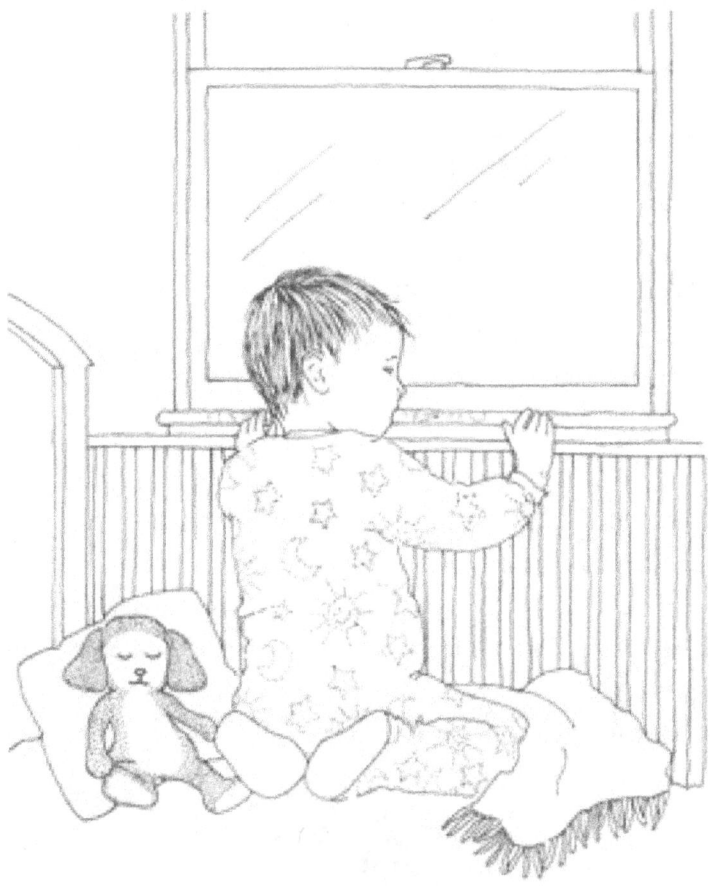

One out of every 40 American children has too much lead in their bodies. The rate of lead poisoning is even higher in cities.

Dust from lead paint is the biggest threat to young children.

Questions to Ask

- Do you live in an older home? Many older homes have lead-based paint or lead water pipes. Lead paint was banned in 1978. Homes built before 1950 are most likely to have lead in paint and water pipes.

- Is there cracking, chipping, or flaking paint in your home?

- Are there places where paint is being rubbed, such as on a door or in a window frame? This can make dust that has lead in it.

- Do you have water pipes made with lead or joined with lead solder? Water that flows through them may contain lead. Lead pipes are dull gray and scratch easily with a key or penny.

- Has your home been recently remodeled or renovated? Projects may leave dust or paint chips with lead.

- Is there lead in the soil outside your home? It may have gotten there from paint on the outside of the building or from industry. Or it may have come from car exhaust from the days when gasoline contained lead. Children can be poisoned if they play in soil that has lead in it or if someone tracks the soil inside the home.

- Does someone you live with work where lead is used? Some jobs that might create lead dust are: construction, bridge building, sandblasting, ship building, plumbing, battery making and recycling, car repair, furniture refinishing, and foundry casting. Workers can bring lead dust home on clothing, skin, or shoes.

- Do you have children under age six who have not had a blood test for lead? Young children should be tested for lead. This is especially true if you live in an older home, if your home has recently been remodeled, or if a brother, sister or a playmate has tested high for lead. Ask your doctor to test your children beginning at six months of age, and then every year until age six.

- Have neighbor children or playmates ever had a high blood lead test?

If you answered yes to any of these questions, your children may be at risk for lead poisoning. Look at the Action Steps on the next page to find out what you can do to protect your children's health!

The Blood Test for Lead

- It only takes a small blood sample to tell if your child has lead poisoning.

- Ask your health care provider about testing.

- Lead levels are measured in micrograms per deciliter (µ/dL).
  - *If your child's level is 10 µ/dL or more, it is too high.*
  - *You need to find out how she or he is getting the lead.*

- Your health care provider can help you find out what to do.

ACTION STEPS

Have Your Children Tested for Lead

- This test is often free at local health clinics.

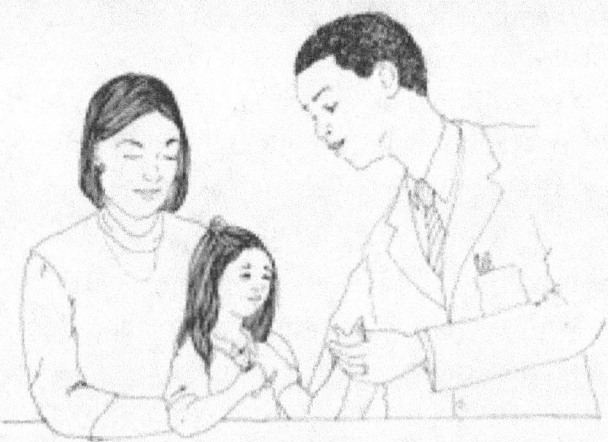

Find Out if Your Home Has Lead

- You may need to have your home or water tested. Your local or state health department can tell you how to do this for little or no cost. Many hardware stores also sell low-cost lead testing kits.

- Don't try to remove lead on your own. It should be done by trained and certified workers. You can find a certified lead paint removal company by contacting your local or state health department. Getting rid of lead in the wrong way can make the problem worse! Children and pregnant women need to stay away during a lead removal project.

Protect Your Children From Lead

- Wash children's hands and face often with soap and water, especially before they eat. Wash toys every week.

- Keep down lead-based paint dust with housekeeping. Wipe windowsills, floors, and other surfaces with paper towels, warm water and soap once a week. Rinse well.

- Never sweep, vacuum, or dry dust in a room that has lead dust. You will not remove the harmful dust and can stir it up. This includes porches, which were often painted with lead paint.

- Don't let children chew or put their mouths on windowsills. Keep cribs away from windowsills and walls.

- If any remodeling is being done, be sure you find out if work is happening on something that contains lead-based paint. Never dry scrape or dry sand lead paint. Don't burn or torch it. Children and pregnant women should stay away while work takes place. Test dust for lead around the remodeling area afterwards.

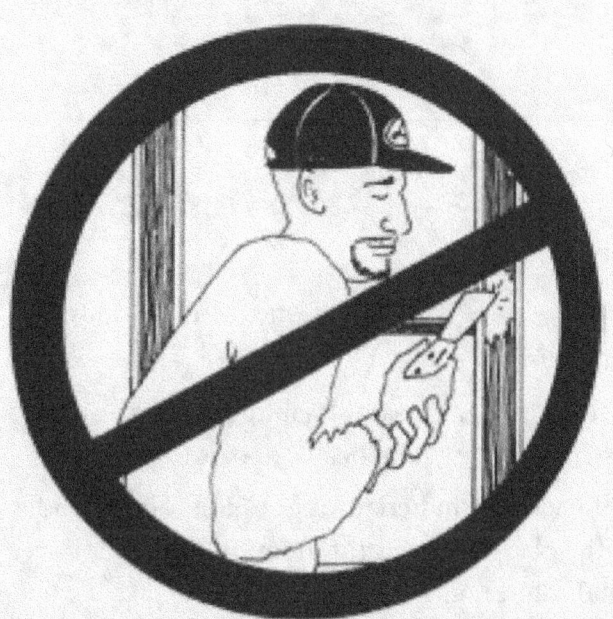

- If you have lead pipes or pipes joined with lead solder, you can take steps to cut down on the lead in your water:

ACTION STEPS, continued

— Never use hot water from the tap for drinking, cooking, or making formula. Hot water can take more lead out of the pipes.

— When you haven't used any water for a few hours or overnight let the cold water run for a few minutes before using it again. You will know it has run long enough when the water changes temperature. Usually it gets colder. This clears out any water sitting in the pipes that may have collected lead or other metals. (See the chapter on drinking water on page 33.)

- Have your water tested for lead. Call your local or state health department to learn how.

- If someone in your home works with lead, they can bring it home on their clothes. Make sure they shower and change clothes and shoes before coming inside. Wash these clothes by themselves.

- If your yard or the yard at your children's daycare may have lead in the soil, don't let your children play there. Have the soil tested for lead to make sure it's safe. Put in grass or other plants to help keep children away from the soil in the meantime.

- Feed your children a healthy diet. Foods with vitamin C, calcium, and iron can help reduce lead poisoning. Children with lead poisoning often don't get enough iron or other minerals in their diets. Making sure your children get enough of these nutrients can lower how much lead their body takes in.

When In Doubt, Check It Out!

- For blood tests, call your family doctor or public health clinic.

- For testing of paint samples and drinking water, call your local or state health department.

- For a packet of materials or questions about lead, call the National Lead Information Center, toll-free at 800/424-LEAD.

- For information on lead in drinking water, call the EPA Safe Drinking Water Hotline: 800/426-4791 or visit the website at www.epa.gov/safewater.

- Contact HUD about tenants' rights and other housing issues at 800/HUDS-FHA—www/hud.gov.

- For more information on Lead In and Around the Home, see *Home*A*Syst*. The *Home*A*Syst* hand book gives more details about this and other healthy home topics. 608/262-0024 or www.uwex.edu/homeasyst.

This chapter was adapted from "Lead In and Around the Home: Identifying and Managing Its Sources," by Karen Filchak, University of Connecticut Cooperative Extension. In *Home*A*Syst*, An Environmental Risk-Assessment Guide for the Home, ©1997 Regents of the University of Wisconsin System. All rights reserved.

Drinking Water

Should You Be Concerned?

Every day Americans drink more than one billion glasses of water! We also depend on water in our homes to clean, cook, fix baby food and formula, and bathe. If you are like most people, you trust that your water is safe. This is mostly true. Public drinking water in the U.S. is safe for most healthy people. If you have a well or other private water supply, it's up to you to keep your drinking water safe. Whether your water comes from a public or private source, you can take steps to make sure it's safe for you and your children.

There are times when your home water supply may not be safe. Using unsafe water to drink or prepare food can make you sick. Children may have more problems than adults because:

- For their size, children drink more than adults.

- Their illnesses may be more serious because children's immune systems are still developing.

- Their bodies are still growing, so chemicals can harm them more.

What May be in Drinking Water that is Not Safe?

Bacteria and viruses can cause diseases. Drinking water with these germs may cause upset stomachs, diarrhea, or more serious illnesses. It can be worse for children, pregnant women, and sick or older people. Just one drink of water with these germs can make you sick.

Nitrate gets into water from animal and human waste, and from fertilizer. Too much nitrate in your drinking water can cause *blue baby syndrome* in babies under six months old. Babies with this problem often have blue or purple-colored faces because they do not get

enough oxygen in their blood. They need to see a doctor right away. Some experts believe nitrate may also result in birth defects and miscarriages. Baby food or formula made with your drinking water needs to be safe.

Lead and copper are metals that can get into water from your pipes. Too much lead can cause children to have learning and behavior problems, and other illnesses (See pages 29-32 for more information on lead). Babies who get too much copper can have colic and spit up their formula more than normal. Older children and adults may get upset stomachs or diarrhea from copper.

Other harmful chemicals can get into drinking water. Pesticides may get into your water supply by washing off lawns and fields or leaking from storage containers. Gas or oil can seep into the ground and get into drinking water. Even very small amounts of some chemicals can cause problems, such as damage to kidneys, liver, or other organs. Some cause cancer and others can cause problems if you are pregnant.

Answer the questions on the next pages to find out if your water is safe and what you can do to cut down on risks to your family.

Questions to Ask

ACTION STEPS

Where Does Your Water Come From?

Does your water come from a public water supply, such as the water utility in your city or town? Or do you have a private water supply, such as a well or spring? The questions to ask yourself depend on where your water comes from.

Public Water Supplies

Before reaching your home, water from a public water supply is tested for over 80 different chemicals. If there are problems, the utility has to treat the water to make it safe or tell you that the water is unsafe to drink.

Every year, water utilities give the results of these water tests to customers. They mail reports or print them in a local newspaper. You can also call your water utility to ask what chemicals are found in the water and how they treat it to make it safe.

Public water can become unsafe after it gets to your home through lead or copper pipes. What kind of pipes do you have?

Lead Pipes: Your home, especially if it is older, may have lead water pipes or pipes joined with lead solder. Lead pipes are dull gray and scratch easily with a key.

Copper Pipes: You may have copper pipes. These are reddish-brown in color.

Clear the Pipes—*Follow this simple step if lead or copper are problems in your home.*

When you haven't used your water for a while (like when you wake up in the morning or when you get home from work), you need to clear out the pipes. Let the cold water run for two or three minutes or until you feel the temperature change, before you drink it or use it for cooking. This will flush out water that has sat in the pipes and picked up lead or copper. Never use hot water from the tap for cooking, drinking, or making formula because the heat helps dissolve the metals faster. Use cold water and heat it on the stove or in the microwave.

Help Protect Water Supplies

You may not know it, but the public water supply is local. Your water may come from the groundwater that is under your home. It may come from the river or lake nearby. What you do can help keep it clean or pollute it.

- If you use poisons to kill bugs or weeds, follow what the label says. Never use more than the label says.

- Watch where you store chemicals (such as bleach, paint, or pesticides) outside. Make sure that the bottles are closed tightly and have labels that say what they are.

- Do not throw chemicals in the garbage or down the drain. Read the label for disposal instructions. Give leftovers to someone who will use them or call your local or state health department to find out how to get rid of them.

ACTION STEPS, continued

- Clean up after your dog. Don't leave pet waste on the ground where rain can wash the germs into rivers and lakes. It's best to flush it down the toilet.

Private Water Supplies

You may have a private water supply, such as a well, for your drinking water. Your well is your responsibility. You need to make sure it is clean and safe.

Test Your Well Water

Has it been more than two years since your water was tested? You cannot see, smell, or taste most problems so you need to have your water tested at a laboratory. Well water is usually tested for bacteria and nitrate. You may want to have your water tested more often or for other pollutants, like pesticides, if you have had problems in the past. Call your local or state health department to find out how to have your water tested.

Protect Your Water Supply

You also need to take care of your well, especially if it is old.

A PRIVATE WELL

cap

12"

casing

drill hole

to house

grout

Do you know where your well is?
Find your well. Is it uphill from animal pens, manure, pet waste, septic systems, dumps, or places where chemicals are stored?

What kind of well do you have?
- A dug or bored well usually has a big hole, two feet across or more, and is less than 50 feet deep. These wells may be less safe because chemicals and bacteria can easily get into the water through the top and sides
- A drilled well usually has a narrow hole (4-10 inches around) and is deeper, sometimes hundreds of feet.
- A driven point or sand-point well is 1-2 inches around and may not be deep.

If you do not know what kind of well you have, contact a local well driller. You can find one in the telephone book.

Do you know how old your well is?
If it is more than 20 years old it may need a checkup. You may need to test your water more often.

Is your well in good shape? You want to keep things from above ground out of your water supply.

ACTION STEPS, continued

- The well casing needs to stick up above the ground, up to 12 inches but local rules vary. Your local or state health department has the information.

- There should be no gaps or spaces between the well casing and the material or soil around it.

- Make sure the casing does not have holes or cracks.

- Does the well cap fit tightly? Are any openings or vents covered by a screen?

- Be sure there is not a low area near the well where rainwater can collect. Rainwater carrying pollutants can get into well water.

- Don't keep gas, oil, weed killer, or other chemicals in your well house.

Do you have unused wells on your property?
Unused wells that have not been properly filled and capped can let pollution into groundwater and make your drinking water unsafe. If you have an unused well, ask your local or state health department how to seal it.

Use devices on the ends of faucets to keep water from flowing back into your water supply. These are called *back flow prevention devices.* They help keep pollutants from washing back into the hose and into your drinking water.

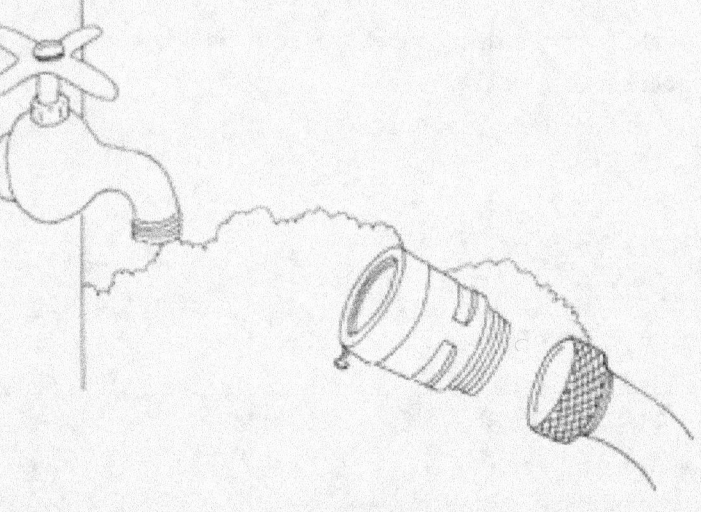

What kind of pipes do you have?
See the section on "Clear the Pipes" on page 34 to find out how to make sure harmful metals are not getting into your drinking water from your pipes.

95% of people living in rural areas drink water from private sources.

When In Doubt, Check It Out!

- Your local water company

- Your local Cooperative Extension office

- Your local or state health department

- EPA's Safe Drinking Water Hotline toll-free at 800/426-4791

- The *Home*A*Syst* handbook gives more details about this and other healthy home topics. 608/262-0024—www.uwex.edu/homeasyst

Notes

This chapter was adapted from "Drinking Water Well Management", by Bill McGowan, University of Delaware Cooperative Extension. In *Home*A*Syst*, An Environmental Risk-Assessment Guide for the Home, ©1997 Regents of the University of Wisconsin System. All rights reserved, and "Your Guide to Public Water", by Alyson McCann, University of Rhode Island Cooperative Extension, February 2000, Rhode Island *Home*A*Syst* program.

Hazardous Household Products

Should You Be Concerned?

Do you have these products in your home? Bleach, rat poison, mothballs, charcoal lighter fluid, oven cleaner, batteries, mercury thermometers, gas, oil, wood polish, toilet and drain cleaners, shoe polish, bug spray?

Household products like these are dangerous for your children!

Household products are called hazardous if they can harm people when not used in the right way. Not every product is hazardous and some are more dangerous than others.

You can use most products safely if you follow the directions on the label. Doing things that are not on the label is risky for your health and your family's. People run into trouble by using too much of a product, or by mixing two products together, for example.

Children can be poisoned if products are stored or thrown away unsafely. Children's bodies are small, so even a little bit of some chemicals can cause big problems.

Eating or drinking a hazardous product is dangerous, of course. Also, just touching or breathing some products—even a very small amount of them—can be harmful. They can burn your skin or eyes just by touching them. Some hazardous products can make you sick if they get into your body through your skin or when you breathe in their dust or fumes.

Sometimes you know right away if you or your child has come into contact with a hazardous product. You may feel sick to your stomach or dizzy. Your skin may itch or burn. Your eyes may water or hurt.

Other problems don't show up until later, like cancer or harm to your lungs. Also, coming into contact with chemicals can affect a child's growing body.

You can protect your children and yourself from illness and injury. Use hazardous products safely. Store them carefully. Dispose of them properly. *The following pages will help you learn more.*

FACT

In 2000, nearly 20,000 children were exposed to or poisoned by household chlorine bleach.

In Case of Emergency

You can reach your local Poison Control Center by calling 1-800-222-1222 from anywhere in the country. Put this number next to all of your telephones and where you store your hazardous products.

Hazardous Household Products

Questions to Ask

Use Safely

Do you use hazardous household products safely?

- Read the label. That is one of the most important steps in using products.

- Look for words like **caution**, **warning**, **flammable**, **harmful, danger, poison**. These tell you that a product may be hazardous. If you see these words on a label, take extra care.

- Look for special instructions on the label such as: "Work in well ventilated area." This means work outside or with the windows open. The fumes can make you sick if you do not have enough fresh air.

- "Wear protective clothing." This means wear goggles or safety glasses, gloves, long sleeves, or other coverings. The right clothing can prevent burns or keep chemicals from going into your body through the skin.

- Never mix products unless the label says it is safe to do it. For example, never mix products containing chlorine bleach with products containing ammonia. You will make a deadly gas by mixing these together.

- Keep children and pets away while you use hazardous products.

- Always put the cap back on and put away the product right after you finish using it.

- Never leave the product or container where children can see it or reach it.

- Don't eat, drink, or smoke when using hazardous products.

- Be ready in case there's an accident: Put the Poison Control Center telephone number, 800/222-1222, where you can find it quickly in case of an emergency. Tape it to the wall by your kitchen phone, for example.

- Buy *Syrup of Ipecac* at your local drugstore and keep it handy. This medicine makes a person throw up. But only use it when a doctor or the Poison Control Center tells you. Sometimes throwing up makes the poisoning worse.

Use Less

Can you cut down on the hazardous products in your home?

- Do you buy only what you need, so you don't have extras?

- Prevent or reduce pest problems so you don't need chemicals to kill them. Wash dishes and wipe counters often. Keep the garbage area tidy.

- If you're pregnant, don't use hazardous products if something else will do the job.

- Think about using tools or products known to be safe: Use a plunger to unclog sinks instead of chemicals. Clean with baking soda (for scrubbing) or vinegar (for cutting grease).

Hazardous Household Products

Questions to Ask

Store Safely

Do you store hazardous household products safely?

- Keep them away from children. A locked, secure place is best.

- Store them in the package, can, or bottle they came in. Never put them in another container (especially one for food or drink)! This helps prevent poisoning and keeps the label instructions with the product.

- Keep containers and packages dry. Close them tightly.

- Set containers inside a plastic bucket in case of leaks.

- Store products at least 150 feet away from your well, cistern, or water pump. This will protect your water supply and your health.

- Keep products away from heat, sparks, or fire.

- Store batteries and flammable chemicals like gasoline in the shade, away from direct sunlight.

Safe Disposal

How do you get rid of leftover products?

- Share the extra with someone who will use it up.

- Take leftovers to a community hazardous waste collection point. Ask your local or state health department where this is.

- Some products—like pesticides—are very hazardous. You will even need to be careful how you dispose of the container. The label will tell you what to do.

- Never dump or burn hazardous products on your property. Dumping or burning them near a water supply is very dangerous.

- Never burn hazardous wastes in a barrel or stove. Burning may let off toxic gases and make hazardous ash and smoke. And, it's against the law in many states.

- Recycle used motor oil or antifreeze. Many communities have places for you to do this.

- Mercury is a threat to health. Products that have mercury in them are fluorescent bulbs, thermometers, thermostats, and blood pressure meters. Call your local trash department or health department to find out where to recycle products with mercury.

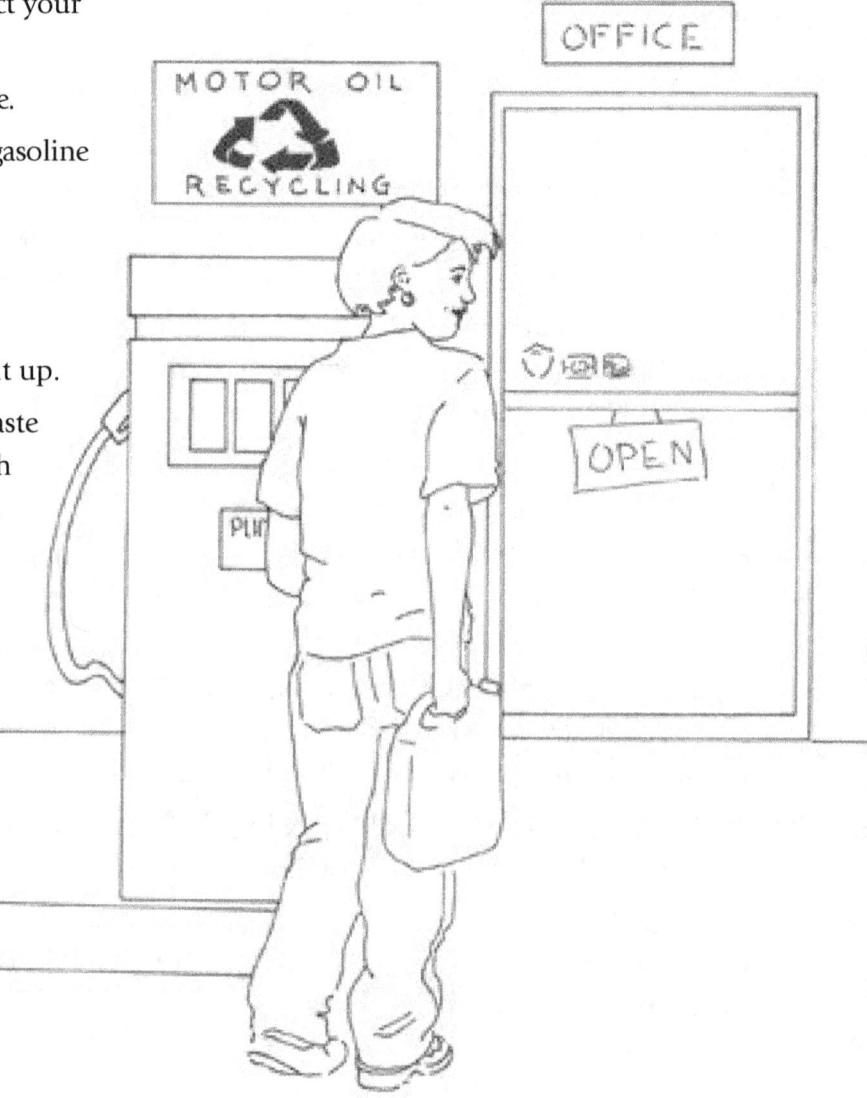

ACTION STEPS

Here are some ways to protect your family's health.

- Buy only what you need to do the job.
- Use products known to be safe when possible.
- Read and follow directions on product labels—always!
- Post the Poison Control Center telephone number next to the phone.
- Never mix two products together unless you are certain it is safe to do so.
- Never mix bleach and ammonia
- Keep all hazardous products, including bleach, in a cabinet out of reach of children.
- Buy products in childproof containers.
- Keep hazardous products in their original containers.
- Give leftover products to someone else to use.
- Find out about your community's hazardous waste collection points.
- Recycle products that you can—oil, antifreeze, products with mercury.
- Never burn or dump leftover products or containers.

Notes

When In Doubt, Check It Out!

- Call your local Poison Control Center 800/222-1222
- Call your local Cooperative Extension office
- Call your local or state health department
- Contact the Consumer Products Safety Commission: 800/638-2772 • www.cpsc.gov
- Contact Healthy Indoor Air for America's Homes: 406/994-3451 or visit the website at www.montana.edu/wwwcxair/
- The *Home*A*Syst* handbook gives more details about this and other healthy home topics 608/262-0024 or www.uwex.edu/homeasyst
- EPA's Consumer Labeling Initiative www.epa.gov/opptintr/labeling/index.htm

This chapter was adapted from "Managing Hazardous Household Products," by Elaine Andrews, University of Wisconsin Cooperative Extension. In *Home*A*Syst*, An Environmental Risk-Assessment Guide for the Home, ©1997 Regents of the University of Wisconsin System. All rights reserved.

Pesticides

Should You Be Concerned?

Many families are bugged by pests. Cockroaches, flies, rats, and mice carry disease and can get into food. Roaches and house dust mites can make allergies and asthma worse. Fleas and ticks riding into the home on pets or clothing can carry disease. The bites of rats and certain spiders can make children and others very ill.

Pesticides are things like bug spray, pet flea collars, rat poison, and garden weed killer that can prevent and kill pests. Pesticides can pose a real danger if you do not use them in the right way. Some may cause poisoning, birth defects, nerve damage, and even cancer. They can make allergies or asthma worse. Breathing fumes or dust from pesticide powders and sprays can be harmful. Touching a floor where pesticide was used can also be dangerous.

Children are especially at risk. When they crawl and play on floors and lawns, they can come into contact with any pesticides used there. Young children put their hands, toys, and other things in their mouths. They may have touched pesticides on the floor or grass.

The biggest danger is poisoning. Children can accidentally poison themselves if they play with, eat, or drink pesticides that are not stored safely.

Almost one-half of homes with a child under five have pesticides stored within reach of children.

POISONED BY CHEMICALS: Don't let this happen to your child

- **A five-year old boy** drinks from a bottle of bleach that he found under the bathroom sink.
- **A three-year old girl** tries to spray her hair the way Mommy does, but sprays an aerosol disinfectant in her eyes instead.
- **A baby** who has just begun to crawl eats green pebbles from behind the sofa. They look like candy but are really rat poison.

The good news is there are lots of things you can do to protect your family's health and safety. Ask yourself the questions on the following page to see if pesticides may be a threat in your home. Safe pesticide use depends on you!

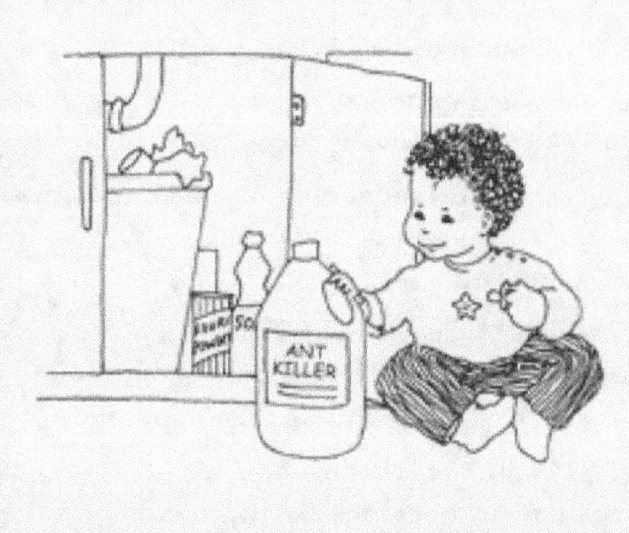

Questions to Ask

Why Do You Have Pests?

- Does your home have loose or torn screens or broken windows?
- Are there gaps or holes in the building that could let in pests?
- Are counters and floors sometimes dirty? Do dishes go unwashed?
- Is there spilled food anywhere in your home?
- Do you keep your garbage where ants, roaches, rats, mice, or other animals can get into it?
- Does your plumbing or roof leak?
- Do you store food in containers or boxes that don't have covers?

Do You Use Pesticides Properly?

Never take it for granted that a pesticide is harmless.

- Do you (or a pest control company) ever use airborne pesticides like flea bombs or roach sprays indoors instead of baits? Bombs and sprays spread pesticides over a larger area, making it more likely someone will come into contact with them.
- Do you use flea collars, sprays, or powder on your pets? These contain pesticides that may harm people.
- Do you use pesticides without reading the label?
- Are children or pets in the room when you use pesticides?
- Do you eat, drink, or smoke while using a pesticide?
- Do you use care when you put bug repellant on your children?
- Do you serve fruits and vegetables without washing them well?

How Do You Store and Dispose of Pesticides?

- Do you ever store pesticides in containers other than the package they came in?
- Do you sometimes have extra, leftover pesticides around the home?
- Do you store pesticides where children can reach them?
- Do you keep pesticides near food?
- Do you throw empty pesticide containers away without rinsing them?
- Do you leave empty pesticide containers where children can reach them?

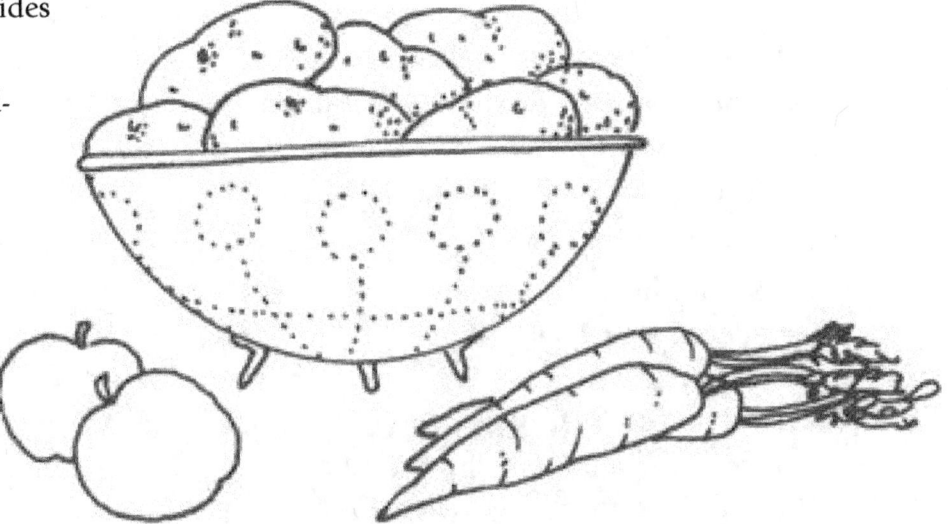

ACTION STEPS

Keep a Clean Home

- Wash children's hands, bottles, pacifiers, and toys often. Regularly clean floors, windowsills, and other surfaces.

- Keep a tight lid on trashcans and empty them often.

- Store food in tightly sealed containers.

- Make sure people in your home eat at the table. Don't let them walk around with food.

- Wipe up spills and crumbs right away.

- Clean up dirty dishes right after eating.

- Clean your home well after treating for roaches to reduce roach allergies.

- Pests need water. Keep them from getting it by fixing leaks and not leaving dishwater in the sink overnight.

- Control fleas by washing bedding often, shampooing pets, vacuuming floors, and using flea combs and traps.

- Get rid of stacks of newspaper, papers, bags, and cardboard boxes that make good homes for pests. Recycle them if you can.

Keep Pests Out of Your Home

- Seal cracks and crevices where pests can get in your home.

- Check things like bags and boxes for roaches before bringing them inside.

- Teach your children not to share combs, hats, or coats at school or daycare.

Use Pesticides Safely

- Read the label and follow the instructions. Use only the amount directed and for the purpose listed.

- Place all pesticides, including baits, out of the reach of children.

- When using a pesticide, keep children away until it has dried or for the time the label recommends.

- Protect your skin, your eyes, and your lungs while using pesticides.

- Always wash your hands after use. Never smoke, eat, or drink while using a pesticide.

- Look for signal words. All pesticide labels include words such as **Caution**, **Warning**, or **Danger** to warn you about a product's hazards.

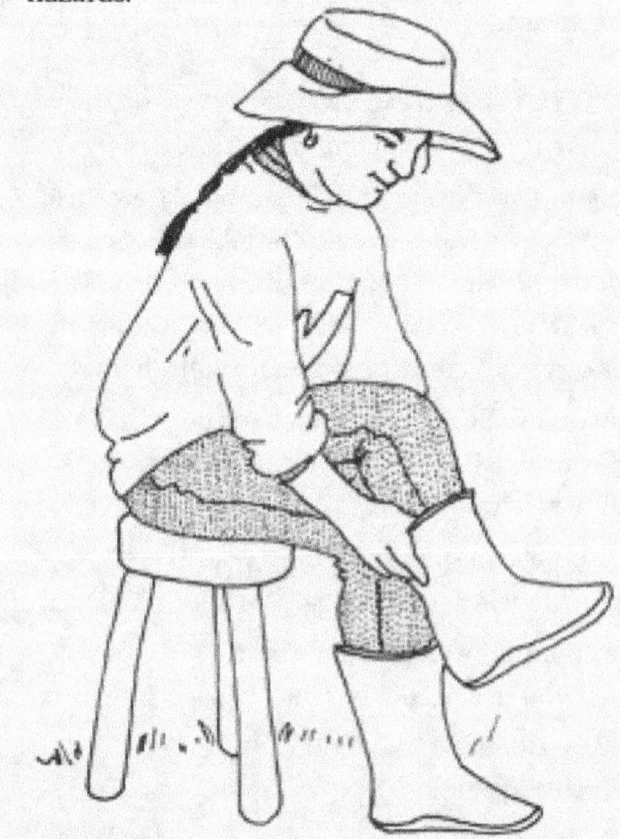

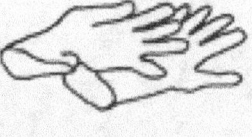
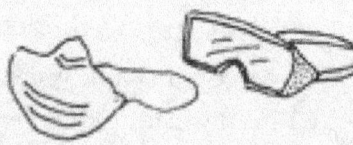

ACTION STEPS, continued

- Wash clothing you wore while using a pesticide in a separate load from other laundry.

- If you have questions about using a pesticide, call the company that made it. An 800 number should be on the label. You can also call the National Pesticide Information Center at 1-800-858-7378.

- Mix and use only the amount you need so you don't have leftovers.

- Mix pesticides outdoors or in an area with plenty of fresh air (Never mix them in the kitchen).

Storing and Disposing of Pesticides

- Store pesticides where children and pets can't reach them or in a locked cabinet.

- Store pesticides only in the container they came in. Never put them in a soft drink bottle or any other kind of container.

- Follow the directions on the label for the right way to throw away pesticides.

- Never use an empty pesticide container for something else.

The word **Caution** shows up on a pesticide label when a product is the least harmful to people.

Warning means a product is more poisonous than one with a Caution label.

Danger means a product is very poisonous or irritating. Use a pesticide that has this word on its label with extreme care because it can burn your skin or eyes very badly.

IN CASE OF EMERGENCY

You can reach your local Poison Control Center by calling 1-800-222-1222 from anywhere in the country.
Put this number next to all of your telephones and where you store your hazardous products.

Bug Repellant

When putting bug repellant on children, read all directions first. Do not use over cuts or broken skin. Do not apply to eyes, mouth, hands, or directly on the face. Use just enough to cover skin or clothing. Don't use it under clothing.

Helpful Tips

Tips For Your Lawn and Garden

- Use lawn seed and plants that grow well in your area and fight disease.

- Think about putting up with a few weeds or insects, rather than using pesticides.

- Use your muscles. You can keep down weeds by hand pulling or hoeing.

- Clean up dead leaves and debris to get rid of homes for pests.

- Make sure you know what the pest or problem is before using a pesticide.

- Use pesticides only where the pests are.

- Your local Cooperative Extension office can help with lawn and garden care.

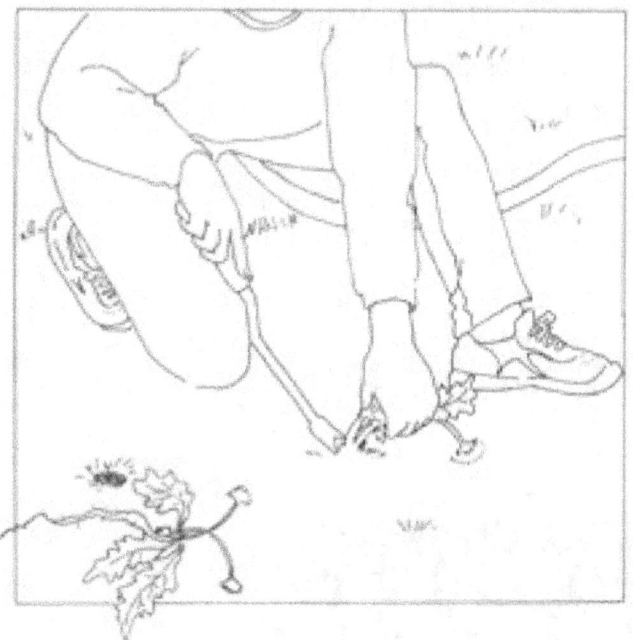

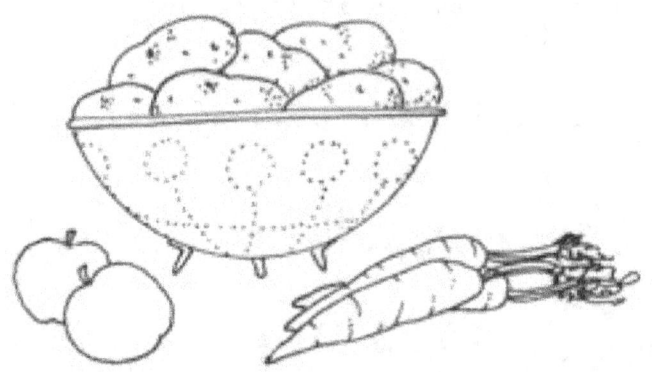

Tips For Preparing Food

- Wash and scrub all fruits and vegetables under running tap water.

- After washing, peel fruits and vegetables when possible.

- Throw away the outer leaves of leafy vegetables like lettuce and other greens.

- Trim fat from meat and skin from poultry and fish—some pesticides collect in fat.

- Eat lots of different foods from lots of different sources.

When In Doubt, Check It Out!

- EPA Office of Pesticide Programs, 703/305-5017
  —www.epa.gov/pesticides
  You can order these publications:

  Help! It's A Roach: A Roach Prevention Activity Book

  Citizen's Guide to Pest Control and Pesticide Safety

  10 Tips to Protect Your Family From Pesticide and Lead Poisoning

  Pesticides and Child Safety

  Pesticides and Food: What You and Your Family Need to Know

- National Pesticide Information Center
  800/858-7378—www.npic.orst.edu

- Food and Drug Administration Food Safety Information Service Hotline, 888/SAFE-FOOD (888/723-3366), 10 a.m. to 4 p.m. Monday through Friday

- The *Home*A*Syst* handbook gives more details about pesticides and other healthy home topics. 608/262-0024—www.uwex.edu/homeasyst

- For more information on non-toxic pest control contact the Bio-Integral Resource Center 510/524-2567—www.birc.org

Notes

This chapter was written by Kadi Row, University of Wisconsin Cooperative Extension. ©2002 University of Wisconsin Extension. All Rights Reserved.

Should You Be Concerned?

Did you know that your chances of getting hurt at home are much higher than they are at work or school? The leading causes of death in the home are falls, drowning, fires, poisoning, suffocation, choking, and guns. The good news is that there are simple steps you can take to protect yourself and your family. This section will help you ask questions to find out if your home is a safe place to live and how to make it even safer.

Very young children and older adults are the most likely to get hurt at home. Keep people's age in mind when thinking about how to keep your home safe.

Falls kill more people than any other type of accident beside car crashes. Most falls happen at home. Most people trip and fall at floor level, not going up or down stairs. Falls can be worse for adults than for children. They fall faster and harder than children. Their bones are weaker, so they break more easily too.

In the U.S., more than one million children age five and under are poisoned each year.

Young children are curious and get into everyday things that can hurt or even kill them. More of them become sick or die from eating or drinking common items like medicine, makeup, and plants. Children like to play with these things because they can look or smell good.

For over a decade, the number of people who die in fires has gone down. Yet fires are still one of the main causes of death in the home. Older adults are most at risk because they may not be able to respond to an alarm or get out of a building quickly.

Choking and suffocation also cause many deaths in the home. When a person chokes, something like a piece of food has gotten stuck in their throat and stopped their breathing. Suffocation happens when a person's nose, mouth, or throat is blocked and they can't breathe. If someone stops breathing long enough they can suffer brain damage or die. Children under age four and older adults are the most likely to die from choking. People can choke on food, or something not meant to be eaten at all, like a button or a coin. Sheets, blankets, and plastic bags can suffocate people who get caught in them.

Drowning kills more than 1,000 children ages 14 and under each year. For every child who drowns, another 20 children go to the hospital or emergency room because they almost drowned.

It takes just a few easy, fairly low-cost steps to keep your children safe from many everyday dangers. The questions below and on the next page will help you find safety problems at home. Page 51 will give you ideas about what to do. Remember, making your home safer for everybody may mean taking more than one step.

Questions to Ask

Slips, Trips, and Falls

- Do you keep your floors—especially hallways and stairs—free of things that might make people slip or trip?
- Are your stairs in good shape?
- Are there throw rugs in your home?
- Do you know the safe way to carry big loads?
- Is your home well lighted?

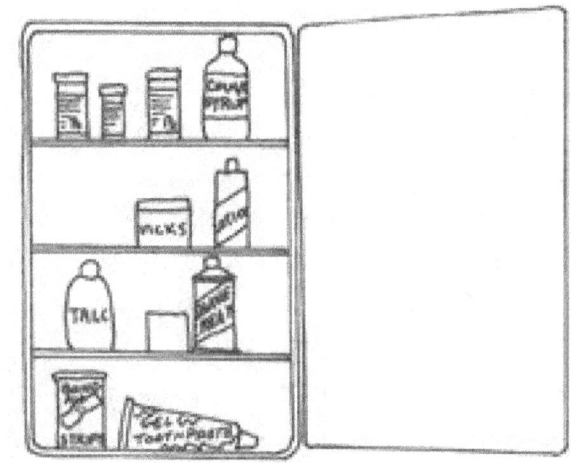

Is Your Home Poison-Proof?

To poison-proof your home, look through each room through the eyes of a child. Is anything that can hurt your child within her or his reach?

Any room can have something in it that can hurt a child: the kitchen, bathroom, bedrooms, living room, basement, garage, or laundry room. Most poisonous products are where people keep cleaning supplies. (See the chapters on Hazardous Household Products page 38 and Pesticides page 42 for more information.)

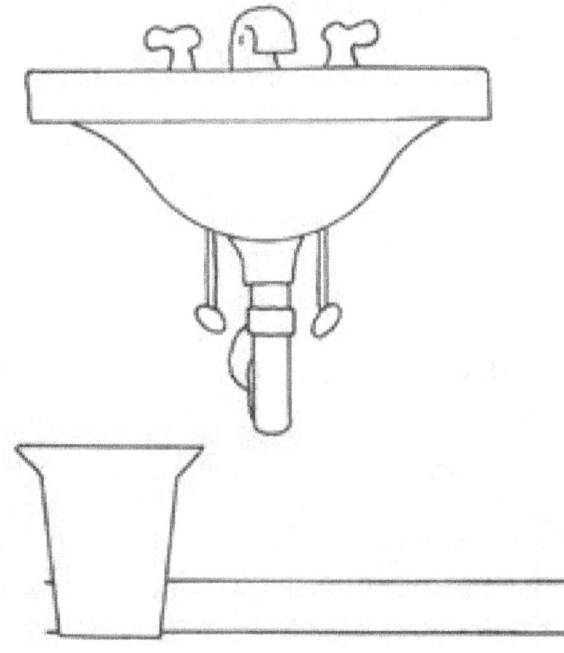

Questions to Ask

Fires and Burns

- Does your house or apartment have at least one smoke alarm?

- Where do you store matches and lighters?

- Have you talked about fire safety with your children?

- Do you have a fire exit plan in case your home catches fire?

- Do you use space heaters safely and with a window open?

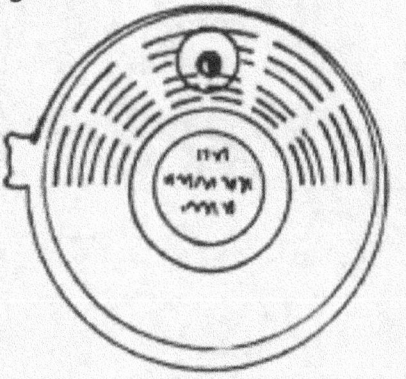

Carbon monoxide is deadly gas you can't see or smell. It comes from combustion appliances like gas heaters, furnaces, stoves or dryers. Car exhaust also has carbon monoxide. See the chapter on carbon monoxide on page 23 to learn how to protect your family from this hidden danger.

To protect your family, put in a carbon monoxide alarm!

Choking

- Do you keep a close eye on young children at meals and at playtime?

- Do you pick out toys that are right for your child's age?

Young children like to put things in their mouths. Balloons, toys, and toy parts that are small enough to fit into a child's mouth may cause choking. You also may not be able to get them out if they get stuck.

Watch Out Around Water

- Do you have a pool or does your child go swimming a lot?

- Does the pool you use have a fence around it?

- Do you ever leave toys in the pool?

- Does your child run around the pool?

- Do you ever visit lakes, beaches, or rivers?

- Do you watch your young children in the bathtub?

Pools are very dangerous for infants and toddlers. A toddler who falls in may die or get brain damage. Toddlers love to play in the water. But they don't know that even shallow water can hurt or kill them. Running children can fall down and hurt themselves badly. Children need to be watched around water at all times.

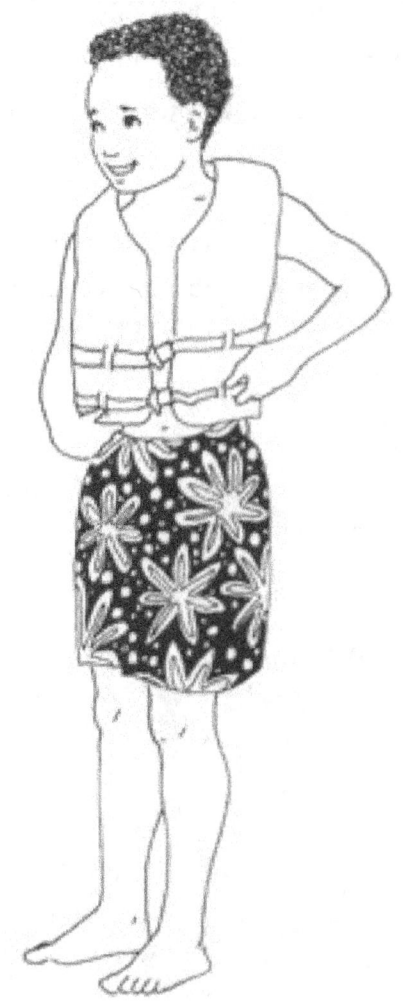

ACTION STEPS

Prevent Slips, Trips, & Falls

- Keep your floors clear of anything that may cause tripping. Pick up hazards such as toys, shoes and magazines.

- Clean up spills right away so people won't slip.

- Repair any stairs that are cracked or worn.

- If there are rugs in your home, use non-skid mats and throw rugs.

- When carrying large or heavy loads, make sure you can see where you're going. Ask for help if you need it.

- Keep your home well lit so you can see where you're walking at night.

Other tips

- Don't use chairs or tables as makeshift ladders.

- Wear shoes with non-skid soles and put young children in non-skid socks.

- Teach your children not to run indoors or jump down stairs.

- Teach your children and other family members about the dangers of falling and how to stay safe.

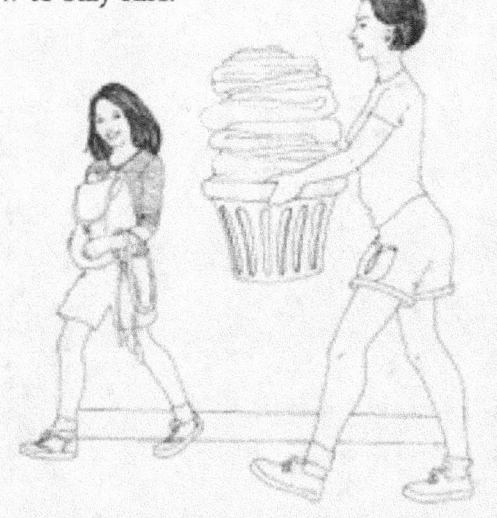

Poison-Proof Your Home

Use this guide to poison-proof your home room-by-room:

- **Kitchen**
  Your kitchen is one of the most dangerous places for a child. Drain openers, detergents, oven cleaners, and other cleaners can hurt you and your children. Put safety latches on all cabinets and drawers with harmful products. Even better, put them in a place that children can't reach. Children often get into dangerous products while someone is using them. If you can, keep your children out of the room while you're cleaning.

- **Bathroom**
  Things in your medicine chest—like medicine, makeup, mouthwash, first aid supplies, deodorants and cleaners can hurt children. Keep these out of their reach. Put a safety latch on your medicine chest.

- **Bedroom**
  Keep medicine, medications, perfumes, makeup, and cigarettes out of children's reach.

- **Living Room**
  Things to look for in the living room are: liquor, cigarettes, furniture polish, lamp oil, and some plants. Keep these out of reach.

- **Garage, Basement, and Laundry Room**
  These are some of the most dangerous places in your home. There are lots of chemicals and poisons in them that can hurt or kill a child: bleach, anti-freeze, gasoline, kerosene, car polishes, car batteries, paints, paint removers, mothballs, bug spray, road salt, and more. It's safest to keep children out of these places altogether.

ACTION STEPS, continued

> **Make sure any medicine is stored in child-safe packaging. But remember, child safe doesn't mean child-*proof*, so keep medicine out of reach.**

Do you know what to do if someone in your home gets poisoned? If you think someone has been poisoned, *call your local Poison Control Center right away at 1-800-222-1222*. Keep this number next to *all* of your telephones. Make sure you know:

- Brand-name of product
- Type of product
- Contents as listed on label
- About how much the person ate or drank
- How the person came in contact with the poison (mouth, skin, etc.)
- How long the person was in contact with the poison
- The person's age and weight
- How you tried to help the person, if you did

Prevent Fires and Burns

Put in a smoke alarm on every floor of your home in or near every sleeping area. This will cut in half the chances of someone dying in a fire.

Playing with fire—matches, lighters, stoves or heaters—is the leading cause of fire-related death for children five and under. Storing matches, lighters, and other heat sources in a safe place like a locked drawer will help keep your children from playing with them. Don't let children play near the stove or grill either.

Teach your children how to prevent fires, and what to do if there is a fire. It can make the difference between life and death. Talk about fire safety with your children. Your local fire department can help.

Plan and practice a fire escape route with your family. Do this at night and with the lights off so you'll be ready if there is a fire. Take special steps for getting children, the elderly, and people who may not be able to save themselves out of the building.

Space heaters such as electric or kerosene heaters cause most burns at home. Keep them out of doorways, halls, or other busy areas. Also, keep them at least three feet from curtains, bedding, or other things that could catch fire. Teach children that heaters will burn. Even better, put up a barrier to keep children and pets away.

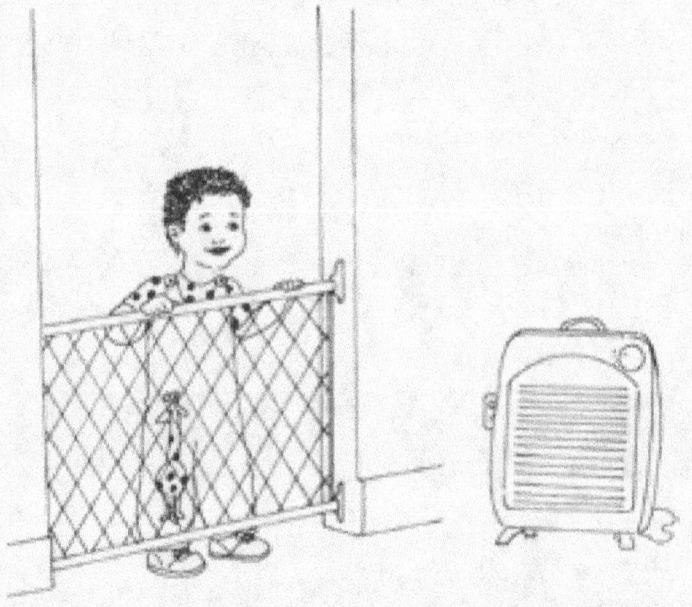

ACTION STEPS, continued

Prevent Choking and Suffocation

Everyday foods can cause choking. Hot dogs, nuts, popcorn, and hard candy can easily get stuck in a small child's throat. Don't let your young children eat them. Even drinks, like formula, milk, or juice can make babies choke if they drink them lying down, especially from a bottle. Make sure children drink sitting up. Keep a close eye on the young children in your home.

Don't let your children play with balloons. Other household items that can cause problems are coins, marbles, and buttons, so keep your floor picked up. Finally, don't let children play near cars or old appliances. They can suffocate and die if they become trapped in a car trunk or old refrigerator.

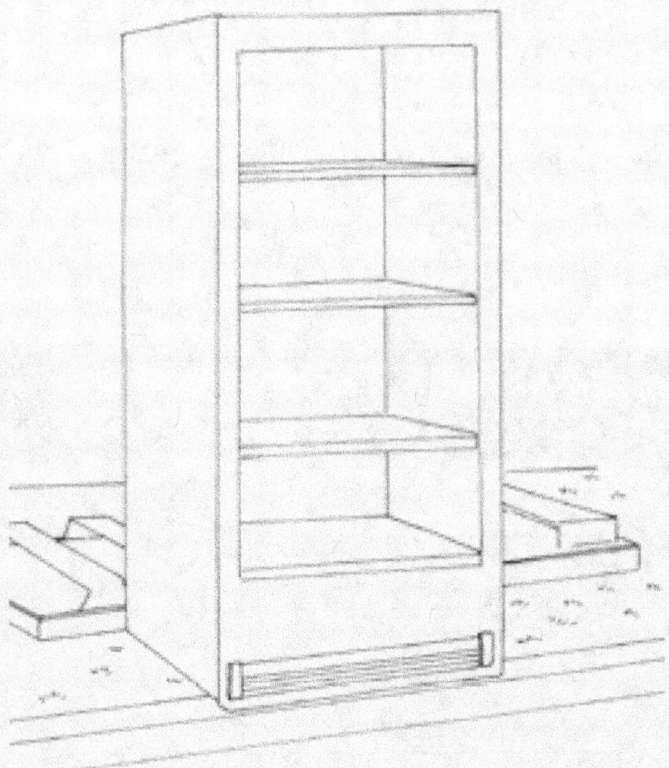

Young children can get tangled up and suffocate in curtains, window blind cords, and extension cords. Plastic bags and covers are also dangerous. Don't tie toys or pacifiers to children's clothes. Very small children should not wear jewelry around their necks.

Toys with small parts or long cords may strangle or cause a child under the age of four to choke. Read a toy's package to make sure it's right for your child.

Watch Out Around Water

If you have or use a pool—Watch children under the age of 12 at all times around pools. Make sure they walk on the pool deck.

All pools, hot tubs, and spas should have a fence at least five feet high, with a self-closing, self-latching gate around them. It's important that this fence be one that children cannot climb. Don't think of your home as part of the fence, because children can open doors to get to a pool.

Take all toys out of the pool area after swimming so children won't go back into the water and play by themselves.

Children should wear life jackets or vests while on docks or at beaches or rivers. Never let a child swim alone!

Never leave a young child alone in the bathtub. Children can drown in only a couple inches of water.

ACTION STEPS, continued

Other Safety Concerns

- Older children and adults should learn first aid and CPR (Cardiopulmonary Resuscitation) so they can help if someone gets hurt. Your local Red Cross offers classes.

- Never let children ride on equipment such as lawn tractors. They may get hurt if they fall off.

- Get safety gear like helmets and kneepads for children riding bicycles, in-line skates, ATVs, scooters, and skateboards. Set a good example by wearing safety gear yourself.

- Store guns safely—unloaded and locked up.

- When traveling by car, make sure that children under 12 ride in the back seat. Use car seats for infants and toddlers under 40 pounds. Use booster seats for children until they are eight years old.

When In Doubt, Check It Out!

- Your local county Extension Office —look in your telephone book

- Your local or state health department —look in your telephone book

- For information on product recalls: The Consumer Products Safety Commission at 800/638-2772 —www.cpsc.gov

- National SAFE KIDS Campaign, 202/662-0600 —www.safekids.org, 1301 Pennsylvania Avenue, NW, Ste. 1000, Washington DC 20004

- The American Red Cross—www.redcross.org

- National Safety Council, 800/621-7619 —www.nsc.org

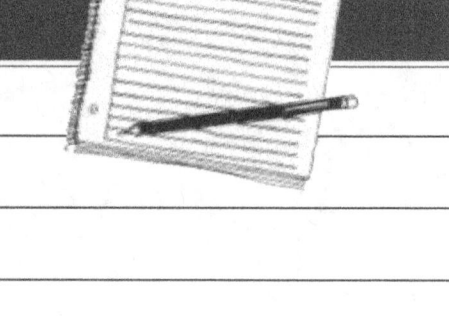

Notes

_____

_____

_____

_____

This chapter was written by Ron Jester, University of Delaware Cooperative Extension. ©2002 University of Wisconsin Extension. All Rights Reserved.

Index

Congratulations!

You have taken the first step toward a safe and healthy home!

*If you have more questions about the health
and safety of your home contact:*

US Department of Housing and
Urban Development:
www.hud.gov/healthyhomes

US Environmental Protection Agency:
www.epa.gov/children/

Children's Environmental Health Network:
www.cehn.org

National Safety Council: www.nsc.org/ehc/
chldhlth.htm

US Centers for Disease
Control and Prevention:
www.cdc.gov/od/oc/childhealth/

Home*A*Syst:
www.uwex.edu/homeasyst

The Lead Listing
www.leadlisting.org